Primary Care ENT

Editors

GRETCHEN DICKSON
RICK KELLERMAN

PRIMARY CARE: CLINICS IN OFFICE PRACTICE

www.primarycare.theclinics.com

Consulting Editor
JOEL J. HEIDELBAUGH

March 2014 • Volume 41 • Number 1

ELSEVIER

1600 John F. Kennedy Boulevard • Suite 1800 • Philadelphia, Pennsylvania, 19103-2899

http://www.theclinics.com

PRIMARY CARE: CLINICS IN OFFICE PRACTICE Volume 41, Number 1
March 2014 ISSN 0095-4543, ISBN-13: 978-0-323-28716-6

Editor: Jessica McCool
Developmental Editor: Yonah Korngold

Primary Care: Clinics in Office Practice (ISSN: 0095–4543) is published quarterly by Elsevier Inc., 360 Park Avenue South, New York, NY 10010-1710. Months of issue are March, June, September, and December. Periodicals postage paid at New York, NY and additional mailing offices. Subscription prices are $225.00 per year (US individuals), $392.00 (US institutions), $115.00 (US students), $275.00 (Canadian individuals), $444.00 (Canadian institutions), $175.00 (Canadian students), $345.00 (international individuals), $444.00 (international institutions), and $175.00 (international students). Foreign air speed delivery is included in all *Clinics* subscription prices. All prices are subject to change without notice. POSTMASTER: Send address changes to *Primary Care: Clinics in Office Practice*, Elsevier Periodicals Customer Service, 11830 Westline Industrial Drive, St. Louis, MO 63146. Customer Service Health Sciences Division, Subscription Customer Service, 3251 Riverport Lane, Maryland Heights, MO 63043. **Customer Service: 1-800-654-2452 (U.S. and Canada); 314-447-8871 (outside U.S. and Canada). Fax: 314-447-8029. E-mail: journalscustomerservice-usa@elsevier.com (for print support); journalsonlinesupport-usa@elsevier.com (for online support).**

Reprints. For copies of 100 or more, of articles in this publication, please contact the Commercial Reprints Department, Elsevier Inc., 360 Park Avenue South, New York, NY 10010-1710. Tel. 212-633-3874; Fax: 212-633-3820; E-mail: reprints@elsevier.com.

Primary Care: Clinics in Office Practice is covered in *MEDLINE/PubMed (Index Medicus)* and *EMBASE/Excerpta Medica, Current Contents/Clinical Medicine, and ISI/BIOMED.*

Printed and bound by CPI Group (UK) Ltd, Croydon, CR0 4YY

Contributors

CONSULTING EDITOR

JOEL J. HEIDELBAUGH, MD, FAAFP, FACG
Clinical Associate Professor, Departments of Family Medicine and Urology, Clerkship
Director, Department of Family Medicine, University of Michigan Medical School,
Ann Arbor; Ypsilanti Health Center, Ypsilanti, Michigan

EDITORS

GRETCHEN DICKSON, MD, MBA
Assistant Professor, Department of Family and Community Medicine, University of Kansas
School of Medicine-Wichita; Program Director, University of Kansas School of Medicine-
Wichita Family Medicine Residency Program at Wesley Medical Center, Wichita, Kansas

RICK KELLERMAN, MD
Professor and Chair, Department of Family and Community Medicine, University of
Kansas School of Medicine-Wichita, Wichita, Kansas

AUTHORS

PATRICK ALLEN, MD
Department of Family and Community Medicine, University of Kansas School of Medicine-
Wichita; Resident, University of Kansas School of Medicine-Wichita Family Medicine
Residency Program at Via Christi Hospitals, Wichita, Kansas

SHERYL BEARD, MD
Clinical Assistant Professor, University of Kansas School of Medicine-Wichita; Senior
Associate Program Director, University of Kansas School of Medicine-Wichita Family
Medicine Residency Program at Via Christi Hospitals, Wichita, Kansas

ALEXI DECASTRO, MD
Assistant Professor, Department of Family Medicine, Medical University of South Carolina;
MUSC Family Medicine Center, Charleston, South Carolina

GRETCHEN DICKSON, MD, MBA
Assistant Professor, Department of Family and Community Medicine, University of Kansas
School of Medicine-Wichita; Program Director, University of Kansas School of Medicine-
Wichita Family Medicine Residency Program at Wesley Medical Center, Wichita, Kansas

JOHN N. DORSCH, MD
Associate Professor, Department of Family and Community Medicine, University of
Kansas School of Medicine-Wichita, Wichita, Kansas

WILLIAM J. HUESTON, MD
Professor, Department of Family Medicine; Senior Associate Dean for Academic Affairs,
Medical College of Wisconsin, Milwaukee, Wisconsin

RICK KELLERMAN, MD
Professor and Chair, Department of Family and Community Medicine, University of Kansas School of Medicine-Wichita, Wichita, Kansas

JOHN M. LASAK, MD
Clinical Assistant Professor, Departments of Surgery and Pediatrics, University of Kansas School of Medicine-Wichita; The Wichita Ear Clinic, Wichita, Kansas

DOUGLAS LEWIS, MD
Clinical Assistant Professor, Department of Family and Community Medicine, University of Kansas School of Medicine-Wichita; Associate Program Director, University of Kansas School of Medicine – Wichita Family Medicine Residency Program at Via Christi Hospitals; Associate Director, Via Christi Adult Cystic Fibrosis Specialty Clinic, Wichita, Kansas

TIM MCVAY, DO
Clinical Assistant Professor, Department of Family and Community Medicine, University of Kansas School of Medicine-Wichita; Associate Program Director, University of Kansas School of Medicine-Wichita Family Medicine Residency Program at Via Christi Hospitals, Wichita, Kansas

LISA MIMS, MD
Instructor, Department of Family Medicine, Medical University of South Carolina, Charleston, South Carolina

DANIEL J. MORGAN, MD
Clinical Instructor, Department of Family and Community Medicine, University of Kansas School of Medicine-Wichita; Hospitalist, Wesley Medical Center, Wichita, Kansas

SCOTT E. MOSER, MD
Professor and Vice Chair for Education, Department of Family and Community Medicine, University of Kansas School of Medicine-Wichita, Wichita, Kansas

HUGH SILK, MD, MPH
Clinical Associate Professor, Department of Family Medicine and Community Health, University of Massachusetts Medical School, Worcester, Massachusetts

RUTH WEBER, MD, MSEd
Clinical Associate Professor, Department of Family and Community Medicine, University of Kansas School of Medicine-Wichita; Associate Program Director, University of Kansas School of Medicine – Wichita Family Medicine Residency Program at Wesley Medical Center, Wichita, Kansas

JENNIFER WIPPERMAN, MD, MPH
Assistant Professor, Department of Family and Community Medicine, University of Kansas School of Medicine-Wichita; Associate Program Director, University of Kansas School of Medicine-Wichita Family Medicine Residency Program at Via Christi Hospitals, Wichita, Kansas

Contents

> Acute otitis externa (AOE) is most often infectious in origin, and can be easily treated with a combination of topical antibiotic and steroid preparations. Systemic antibiotics are rarely needed for AOE. Chronic otitis externa (COE) can be more difficult to treat, but if an underlying cause can be identified this condition can often be successfully managed. In both AOE and COE, prevention is fundamental. If patients are able to avoid precipitating factors, future episodes can often be averted.

> 1 in 4 children will have at least 1 episode of acute otitis media (AOM) by age 10. AOM results from infection of fluid that has become trapped in the middle ear. The bacteria that most often cause AOM are *Streptococcus pneumoniae*, *Haemophilus influenzae*, and *Moraxella catarrhalis*. Differentiating AOM from otitis media with effusion (OME) is a critical skill for physicians, as accurate diagnosis will guide appropriate treatment of these conditions. Although fluid is present in the middle ear in both conditions, the fluid is not infected in OME as is seen in AOM patients.

> Hearing loss may affect all age groups from the newborn to the elderly, impacting speech and language development in children and causing social and vocational problems for adults. Hearing loss can arise from anywhere in the auditory circuit including the external auditory canal, sound conduction mechanism, cochlea, cochlear nerve, and central auditory pathways. Rehabilitation options exist for all types of hearing loss, regardless of cause or location within the auditory system. Awareness of symptoms, signs, and rehabilitative measures aids primary care physicians in early identification and treatment of hearing loss.

> Rhinitis is caused by a variety of allergic and nonallergic mechanisms. Mild disease can usually be managed with avoidance measures alone. Allergen removal can also improve the severity of allergic rhinitis and can reduce the

need for medications. Allergic rhinitis is represented by sneezing, nasal congestion, nasal pruritus, and rhinorrhea. Oral antihistamines should be used to treat patients with mild or occasional seasonal allergic rhinitis. Because of the variance in causes of nonallergic rhinitis, treatments also vary. Irrigation and debridement are the standard treatment of atrophic rhinitis. For gustatory rhinitis, pretreatment with ipratropium bromide can be used.

Rhinosinusitis

Alexi DeCastro, Lisa Mims, and William J. Hueston

Although sinusitis is common, controversy exists regarding terminology, diagnostic criteria, indications for imaging, and treatment guidelines. Patients who are diagnosed with bacterial sinusitis should be started on amoxicillin-clavulanate unless an allergy to penicillin is reported, in which case doxycycline or a respiratory fluoroquinolone is indicated for nonpregnant patients. Patients who fail to respond to antibiotic therapy should be suspected of having chronic sinusitis, which may require additional therapy, including endoscopic surgery. Referral of these patients to an otolaryngologist for further evaluation is recommended. Patients with severe systemic symptoms including altered mental status or severe headaches should be suspected of having fungal sinusitis and to an otolaryngologist acutely because this condition has high mortality if not treated emergently.

Epistaxis: Evaluation and Treatment

Daniel J. Morgan and Rick Kellerman

Epistaxis, or nosebleed, is a common disorder that many patients will experience. Most patients go to the emergency room when they have an uncontrolled nosebleed, or they may present to an outpatient office. Most nosebleeds are not life-threatening and can be managed conservatively. Occasionally, hospital admission, referral to an otolaryngologist physician, and/or blood transfusion may be necessary. This article is an update on the latest information related to the prevention, causes, and treatment of epistaxis.

Diseases of the Mouth

Hugh Silk

Oral pathologic abnormality is common and can be potentially serious. There are many diseases of the mouth that medical personnel must be able to diagnose and initiate management. The most prevalent lesions can be categorized as infectious, inflammatory, and common benign and malignant lesions. This article discusses prevalence, cause, diagnosis, and management of lesions such as stomatitis, candidiasis, caries, oral cancers, and bony tori.

Pharyngitis

Ruth Weber

Most infectious pharyngitis has a viral cause. The use of aspirin or nonsteroidal anti-inflammatory agents (NSAIAs) is advised in adults and NSAIAs in children for the treatment of pain. There are several studies that show that NSAIAs relieve pharyngitis pain better than acetaminophen. Penicillin remains the antibiotic of choice of group A beta-hemolytic streptococcal (GAS) pharyngitis. Resistance has not developed to penicillin. Patients with GAS pharyngitis should have improvement in 3 to 4 days. If not better at that time, the patient should be seen for diagnostic reconsideration or the development of a suppurative complication.

PRIMARY CARE: CLINICS IN OFFICE PRACTICE

RELATED INTEREST

Otolaryngologic Clinics of North America, June 2013 (Vol. 46, Issue 3)
Complementary and Integrative Therapies for ENT Disorders
John Maddalozzo, Edmund Pribitkin, and Michael Seidman, *Editors*
Available at: http://www.oto.theclinics.com/

Foreword

Drips, Plugs, and Scratches

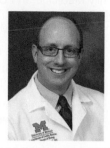

Joel J. Heidelbaugh, MD, FAAFP, FACG
Consulting Editor

"Common" ear, nose, and throat (ENT) issues will always be the mainstay in primary care practices. Cough variants, pharyngitis, and ear pain/otitis perennially rank in the top 20 diagnoses for visits in ambulatory care practices.[1] Clinicians struggle with keeping up on the latest evidence for whether to treat or not to treat these conditions with antibiotics, and when to appropriately refer to an otolaryngologist. These common ENT conditions account for a substantial portion of billing in office and hospital revenue, which translates to large expenditure in ambulatory and emergency department utilization and resources. While many ENT issues require office evaluation, a significant percentage can also often be triaged effectively over the phone with appropriate protocols, while some more emergent conditions require prompt evaluation.

It's amazing how many of these conditions I see in my daily practice, and how chronic many of them have become in both children and adults: recurrent otitis, recurrent strep pharyngitis, chronic epistaxis, unexplained dizziness and vertigo, and the commonly overlooked cases of hearing loss. The phone-call requests for "drippy noses," "plugged ears," and "scratchy throats" are all very frequent and seasonally predictable. I continue to be baffled at the myths behind "teething doesn't lead to ear infections," "I need antibiotics when I get a sore throat because it's always strep," and "my previous doctor always just gave me antibiotics for my cough." We remain challenged and often ill-equipped with the knowledge of how to approach the patient with dizziness and vertigo. So what do we do?

This issue of *Primary Care: Clinics in Office Practice* details diseases of the inner and outer ear, including dizziness, vertigo, and hearing loss; oropharyngeal diseases and disorders; common rhinosinusitis conditions; and includes an overview on neurologic syndromes of the head and neck. I would like to congratulate Drs Dickson and Kellerman, as well as the talented authors of this issue, on a phenomenal accomplishment. A publication as unique as this one deserves special recognition, on account of

Prim Care Clin Office Pract 41 (2014) ix–x
http://dx.doi.org/10.1016/j.pop.2013.10.013   **primarycare.theclinics.com**
0095-4543/14/$ – see front matter © 2014 Elsevier Inc. All rights reserved.

both its practicality and its comprehensiveness. This compendium of articles is a must-read for primary care clinicians at every level.

Joel J. Heidelbaugh, MD, FAAFP, FACG
Departments of Family Medicine and Urology
University of Michigan Medical School
Ann Arbor, MI, USA

Ypsilanti Health Center
200 Arnet Suite 200
Ypsilanti, MI 48198 USA

E-mail address:
jheidel@umich.edu

REFERENCE

1. Centers for Disease Control and Prevention. FastStats–Ambulatory Care Use and Physician Visits. Available at: http://www.cdc.gov/nchs/fastats/docvisit.htm. Accessed October 25, 2013.

Preface

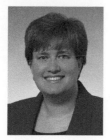 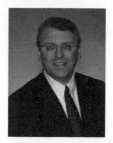

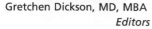

Gretchen Dickson, MD, MBA   Rick Kellerman, MD
Editors

Hardly a day goes by in a busy primary care office where a physician does not encounter a condition of the ears, nose, or throat. Ranging from the minor, common conditions of childhood to rare, life-changing ailments, the primary care physician must be ready to appropriately diagnose, confirm, and treat patients for this myriad of pathologic abnormality. The articles of this issue focus on the common conditions that will likely be encountered in a primary care office, such as otitis media, Group A streptococcal pharyngitis, and epistaxis. We have included articles on common concerns that can stymie primary care physicians, such as dizziness and oral lesions. In addition, there is information on rare yet disabling conditions, such as facial neuralgias. It is our hope that you find this issue informative and practical for use in a busy office.

Gretchen Dickson, MD, MBA
Department of Family and Community Medicine
University of Kansas School of Medicine-Wichita
1010 North Kansas Street
Wichita, KS 67214, USA

Rick Kellerman, MD
Department of Family and Community Medicine
University of Kansas School of Medicine-Wichita
1010 North Kansas Street
Wichita, KS 67214, USA

E-mail addresses:
gdickson@kumc.edu (G. Dickson)
RKELLERM@kumc.edu (R. Kellerman)

Prim Care Clin Office Pract 41 (2014) xi
http://dx.doi.org/10.1016/j.pop.2013.10.014
0095-4543/14/$ – see front matter © 2014 Elsevier Inc. All rights reserved.

Otitis Externa

Jennifer Wipperman, MD, MPH

KEYWORDS

- Acute otitis externa • Chronic otitis externa • Antibiotics • Topical steroids

KEY POINTS

- Acute otitis externa most often is infectious in origin, and can be easily treated with a combination of topical antibiotic and steroid preparations.
- Systemic antibiotics are rarely needed for acute otitis externa.
- Chronic otitis externa can be more difficult to treat, but if an underlying cause can be identified this condition can often be successfully managed.
- In both acute and chronic otitis externa, prevention is fundamental. If patients are able to avoid precipitating factors, future episodes can often be averted.

Otitis externa is a common problem seen in the primary care office, and most cases are managed by primary care providers.[1] Otitis externa is an inflammatory condition of the external ear canal, with or without infection. Inflammation may be localized to the ear canal, or include portions of the outer ear, such as the pinna or tragus. Acute otitis externa (AOE) is defined as lasting less than 6 weeks, and chronic otitis externa (COE) as lasting 3 months or longer. AOE, also known as swimmer's ear, is usually an infectious condition, whereas COE more often has a noninfectious, allergic cause.

ACUTE OTITIS EXTERNA
Epidemiology

The overwhelming majority (>95%) of otitis externa cases are acute.[2] AOE occurs most often in the summer and in warmer, humid climates. Each year, 1 to 2.5 in 100 people are affected.[1,2] Peak incidence arises among children of age 7 to 12 years, and is 5 times more common in regular swimmers.[3]

Risk Factors

In addition to living in warmer, humid climates and swimming, other risk factors relate to increased moisture in the ear canal, loss of protective cerumen, and trauma to the ear canal.[4] Cerumen impaction can cause water retention in the ear canal and may

Department of Family and Community Medicine, University of Kansas School of Medicine – Wichita, 1010 North Kansas, Wichita, KS 67214, USA
E-mail address: jennifer.wipperman@viachristi.org

Prim Care Clin Office Pract 41 (2014) 1–9
http://dx.doi.org/10.1016/j.pop.2013.10.001
0095-4543/14/$ – see front matter © 2014 Elsevier Inc. All rights reserved.

predispose to AOE. On the other hand, removal of cerumen by excessive cleaning leads to a loss of protective waxy barrier and breakdown of the epithelial lining. Trauma to the ear canal may also occur from use of a hearing aid or ear plug. AOE is more common among those with chronic dermatologic conditions, such as psoriasis or atopic dermatitis, which causes debris and skin breakdown in the ear canal.[5] Finally, those who are immunocompromised, including patients with diabetes mellitus, may have more severe and resistant cases of AOE.[2]

Pathophysiology

The external auditory canal is about 25 mm long and curves in an S-shape toward the tympanic membrane.[4] The outer one-third of the canal base is cartilaginous whereas the inner two-thirds is bony. Hair follicles and cerumen-producing glands cover the outer one-third of the canal. Cerumen has several protective functions in the ear canal. First, it provides a waxy barrier that protects the epithelium from breakdown caused by excessive moisture exposure. Second, cerumen has a slightly acidic pH and lysozymal activity that inhibits bacterial and fungal growth.[6] Disturbance in the normal acidic environment, lack of cerumen, and trauma to the epithelial lining can lead to bacterial or fungal infection of the ear canal, causing an inflammatory response. More than 98% of infectious AOE is bacterial.[3] The most likely pathogens include *Pseudomonas aeruginosa* and *Staphylococcus* spp, and AOE is often a polymicrobial infection. Less often, gram-negative bacteria may be involved. Rarely, AOE may result from a fungal (*Candida* or *Aspergillus*) infection.[7]

Clinical Presentation

Patients with AOE present with the rapid onset of ear pain, fullness, and otorrhea. Pain that is worse with traction on the pinna or palpation of the tragus is the hallmark of AOE. In the initial stages, patients may experience mild discomfort and ear pruritus. On examination, the ear canal may be erythematous and slightly edematous, with minimal discharge. Often the severity of pain experienced by the patient is disproportionate to physical examination findings. As the condition progresses, the canal may become extremely edematous and nearly obstructed from additional otorrhea and debris. Inflammation may spread to the tympanic membrane, causing myringitis. A sensation of ear fullness may occur, as well as hearing loss if obstruction is severe. Regional lymphadenitis and surrounding cellulitis of the pinna may be present. Of importance, systemic symptoms such as fever and malaise suggest extension beyond the ear canal.

Diagnosis

AOE is a clinical diagnosis, the criteria of which are listed in **Box 1**. Diagnosis requires a history of rapid onset (within the last 48 hours) occurring in the last 3 weeks with signs and symptoms of ear canal inflammation.[2] Symptoms include otalgia, itching, or fullness, with or without hearing loss. Signs include tenderness of the outer ear or diffuse ear-canal edema or erythema with or without otorrhea, regional lymphadenopathy, tympanic membrane erythema, or surrounding cellulitis. Several other conditions can mimic AOE, and should be differentiated (**Table 1**).

In uncomplicated cases, obtaining cultures of otorrhea is not necessary. However, bacterial and fungal cultures may be helpful in resistant or recurrent cases in patients with a history of frequent topical antibiotic use or the immunocompromised. If malignant (necrotizing) otitis externa is suspected, cultures should always be obtained.

Pneumatic otoscopy and tympanometry are useful in differentiating AOE from acute otitis media (AOM). This distinction is important because otitis media would require

Box 1
Diagnostic criteria for acute otitis externa

1. Rapid onset (generally within 48 hours) in the past 3 weeks, AND

2. Symptoms of ear canal inflammation that include:

   - Otalgia (often severe), itching, or fullness

   - WITH OR WITHOUT hearing loss or jaw pain, AND

3. Signs of ear canal inflammation that include:

   - Tenderness of the tragus, pinna, or both

   - OR diffuse ear canal edema, erythema, or both

   - WITH OR WITHOUT otorrhea, regional lymphadenitis, tympanic membrane erythema, or cellulitis of the pinna and adjacent skin

Data from Rosenfeld RM, Brown L, Cannon CR, et al. Clinical practice guideline: acute otitis externa. Otolaryngol Head Neck Surg 2006;134(Suppl 4):S4–23.

Table 1
Differential diagnosis of acute otitis externa

Condition	Clinical Characteristics
Carcinoma of the ear canal	May be indistinguishable from otitis externa. Consider if abnormal tissue growth in ear canal, or patients with mild pain, bloody otorrhea, and lack of response to treatment of otitis externa
Chronic suppurative otitis media	Develops after tympanic membrane rupture in acute otitis media. Chronic drainage leads to otalgia, otorrhea, and, possibly, eczematous changes
Contact dermatitis	Often develops after exposure to topical agents such as neomycin, anesthetics, or commercial products. Itching usually present. May see maculopapular rash on conchal bowel and edematous ear canal
Eczema or psoriasis	Patients with history of disorder and/or typical rash present elsewhere on the body. May have ear canal pruritus, hyperkeratosis, and lichenification
Furunculosis	Infection of hair follicle in ear canal manifested by a tender, erythematous papule or pustule
Herpes zoster oticus	Causes vesicles on external ear canal, posterior auricle, and, possibly, tympanic membrane. Patients often have severe otalgia and facial nerve palsy
Malignant otitis externa	Consider in patients with findings of severe otitis externa unresponsive to treatment, granulation tissue in ear canal, and systemic signs such as temperature >38°C
Otomycosis	Patients often experience itching more than otalgia. Fluffy, cotton-like debris may be noted in the ear canal, possibly with hyphae and otorrhea
Seborrheic dermatitis	May see typical seborrhea on face, hairline, and scalp. Ear canal often with minimal cerumen and is flaky, shiny, dry, and erythematous

oral antibiotics of an appropriate regimen. In cases of otitis externa, pneumatic otoscopy will show normal motion of tympanic membrane, and tympanometry will show a normal peaked tracing. On the other hand, in AOM there will be negligible motion of tympanic membrane with pneumatic otoscopy and a flat tracing on tympanometry. If the tympanic membrane is obstructed from canal edema and discharge, tympanometry can be used to determine whether it is intact. In the presence of AOE without AOM, tympanometry will show a normal tracing if the tympanic membrane is intact.

Treatment

The mainstays of treatment for AOE include pain control, treatment of infection, and avoiding precipitating factors. These goals are most often accomplished with aural toilet, a topical antibiotic and topical steroid, and over-the-counter oral pain medication if needed. Oral antibiotics are rarely indicated.

Topical antibiotics are effective for most cases. Most often, an aminoglycoside or fluoroquinolone antibiotic is used, as they include coverage of *Pseudomonas* and *Staphylococcus* spp. An aminoglycoside preparation, as found in Cortisporin Otic, should be avoided if the tympanic membrane is perforated or if the patient has a history of contact sensitivity to neomycin. Up to 15% of the population has contact sensitivity to neomycin, which increases to 30% among those with chronic or eczematous otitis externa.[8,9] Aminoglycosides are ototoxic, and can lead to hearing loss and vertigo if they reach the inner ear.[10] Both aminoglycoside and fluoroquinolone antibiotics have a 70% to 90% clinical response rate.[11] Because topical acetic acid preparations (VoSol) have anti-infective activity and drying action, they exhibit clinical cure rates similar to those of topical antibiotics for AOE.[11] However, acetic acid preparations may be less effective if needed for a longer than 1 week.[12]

A 2010 Cochrane review found no difference in efficacy between classes of antibiotics.[11] Therefore, choice of antibiotic should be based on factors such as risk of ototoxicity, contact sensitivity, availability, cost, dosing schedules, and patient compliance (**Table 2**). Because topical antibiotics reach a high concentration in the ear canal, even bacterial strains considered resistant to systemic antibiotics (ie, methicillin-resistant *Staphylococcus aureus*) are susceptible to topical antibiotic preparations.[2] The addition of a topical steroid results in reduced canal edema and otorrhea, and hastens pain relief.[11,13] Many topical antibiotic preparations include a steroid component. In general, patients should be treated for 7 to 10 days.[2] Practically, patients may be advised to use drops for 1 week. If symptoms are not resolved they may continue to use drops until a few days after symptoms resolve, up to 1 additional week. If symptoms still persist at day 14, this should be considered a treatment failure.

Proper use of topical antibiotics is important, and misunderstanding of technique can lead to treatment failure. For this reason, placement of drops should be taught in the office. Up to 40% of patients do not self-administer drops correctly.[14] Having someone else administer topical preparations is therefore usually more effective. Patients should lie on their side with the affected ear up. Drops should be placed to run along the side of the ear canal until it is filled, gently moving the pinna to and fro to eliminate air trapping and ensure filling. Patients should remain in this position for at least 3 to 5 minutes.

For topical antibiotics to be effective, they must contact the epithelial lining. Therefore, in patients with a significant amount of debris or otorrhea, aural toilet may be necessary. In general, debris can be cleared using gentle suction, irrigation, or dry mopping with cotton. Impacted cerumen and foreign bodies should be removed. Gentle irrigation should be used only if the tympanic membrane is intact, and should

Table 2
Common topical antimicrobial preparations for acute otitis externa

Component	Brand Name	Cost of Generic (Brand)	Dosage	Comments
Acetic acid 2%	VoSol	$30 for 15 mL ($36 for 15 mL)	3–5 drops every 4–6 h	Avoid if tympanic membrane ruptured. May cause local irritation
Acetic acid 2%/ hydrocortisone	VoSol HC	$50 for 10 mL ($50 for 10 mL)	3–5 drops every 4–6 h	As above
Neomycin/ polymyxin B/ hydrocortisone	Cortisporin	$18 for 10 mL ($100 for 10 mL)	3–4 drops every 6–8 h	—
Ciprofloxacin/ hydrocortisone	Cipro HC	Not available ($190 for 10 mL)	3–4 drops every 12 h	7-Day course adequate
Ciprofloxacin/ dexamethasone	Ciprodex	Not available ($160 for 7.5 mL)	3–4 drops every 12 h	As above
Ofloxacin	Floxin Otic	$20 for 5 mL ($80 for 5 mL)	10 drops once daily	7-Day course adequate

Data from GoodRX. Available at: www.goodrx.com. Accessed November 20, 2013.

be avoided in patients with poorly controlled diabetes mellitus or the immunocompromised. Irrigation has been associated with malignant otitis externa.[15]

Ear wicks may ensure adequate antibiotic delivery in patients with marked edema. Wicks are made of compressed cellulose material, and expand when exposed to moisture. This approach facilitates drug delivery and reduces edema.[16] Once a wick is placed, it should be moistened with saline. Edema generally improves within the first few days, after which the wick will fall out spontaneously, or it may be removed by the clinician at a follow-up visit.

For pain control, most patients may use oral over-the-counter medications such as acetaminophen or ibuprofen.[2] As already noted, the addition of a topical steroid hastens pain relief by a median of 1 day compared with topical antibiotics alone. If pain is severe, narcotic pain medications may be necessary. Topical benzocaine preparations are generally best avoided in AOE. Although benzocaine's anesthetic action provides excellent pain relief, it can mask progression of disease. Furthermore, the additional drops can limit penetration of topical antibiotics. Some patients may also develop contact dermatitis from topical benzocaine.[17]

Even though systemic antibiotics are rarely needed in AOE, they continue to be prescribed to one-third of patients with AOE.[18] Frequently the chosen antibiotic is not effective against *Pseudomonas*. Moreover, systemic antibiotics are associated with increased bacterial resistance, side effects, and increased cost. Systemic antibiotics are indicated in patients with surrounding cellulitis of the external ear and beyond, uncontrolled diabetes, the immunocompromised, those with a history of radiation to the head, and those in whom canal edema limits penetration of topical antibiotics.[2]

Finally, patients with AOE should avoid precipitating factors. In general, swimming should be avoided until the infection is resolved, although recreational swimming may be allowed as long as patients do not submerge their head. Competitive swimmers should avoid swimming for 2 to 3 days, or until the pain resolves if they use well-fitting ear plugs. Use of hearing aids and ear plugs should be avoided until symptoms resolve.

Monitoring

Most patients with AOE will experience significant improvement within 24 hours.[16] If patients do not improve within 48 to 72 hours, they should be reevaluated. Clinical failure may be due to nonadherence, inadequate drug delivery, canal obstruction, or misdiagnosis. Although most patients can be treated by their primary care provider, referral is indicated in cases of suspected malignant otitis externa, lack of improvement, or an inability to remove obstructing debris or a foreign body.

Prevention

Patients with AOE should prevent future episodes by limiting predisposing factors. Moisture retention in the ear canal should be minimized, and a healthy skin barrier maintained. Excessive moisture can be avoided in several situations. Swimmers may use well-fitting ear plugs while swimming to prevent water retention in the ear canal. After water exposure, the head should be tilted and the ear gently pulled to empty any residual water. A hair dryer on the lowest heat setting may be used to help dry the ear. In addition, acidifying drops, such as acetic acid 2% (VoSol otic solution) may be placed in the ear after water exposure to dry the ear canal.

Sources of ear trauma should also be avoided. Patients should be instructed to stop frequent ear cleaning, especially with cotton-tipped applicators. Hearing aids should be examined to ensure that they fit well. Underlying dermatologic conditions should be adequately treated.

Complications

In AOE, infection may spread from the ear canal itself to surrounding structures, leading to auricular or facial cellulitis, perichondritis, or chondritis.[4] Ongoing chronic infection may result in canal stenosis and hearing loss.[19]

Malignant (necrotizing) otitis externa is a severe life-threatening complication of AOE.[20] It may occur in untreated cases where infection extends to the temporal bone, causing osteomyelitis and systemic toxicity. *Pseudomonas* is most often implicated. Malignant otitis externa is most common among adult patients, including the elderly, those with diabetes mellitus, and the immunocompromised.[15] Nearly 90% to 100% of patients with malignant otitis externa have diabetes mellitus.[20] Further complications include meningitis, dural sinus thrombosis, cranial abscess, and cranial nerve palsies. Facial nerve paralysis may be seen early during infection.

Malignant otitis externa should be suspected in patients with signs of systemic toxicity, such as fever, or failure to improve with topical antibiotics. In addition to symptoms of severe AOE, patients may also complain of headache, temporal mandibular joint pain, and trismus. On examination, in addition to severe canal edema, erythema, and otorrhea, granulation tissue is often present on the floor of the canal, especially at the bony-cartilaginous junction. Diagnosis is confirmed by imaging with computed tomography or magnetic resonance imaging. Patients will often have an elevated sedimentation rate, and cultures of otorrhea should always be obtained. Treatment requires initial empiric intravenous antibiotics that cover *Pseudomonas*. In severe or resistant cases, surgical debridement may be necessary.

CHRONIC OTITIS EXTERNA

In contrast to AOE, chronic otitis externa (COE) is more often attributed to allergic or autoimmune causes than infectious etiology. Less than 5% of otitis externa is chronic.[2] However, COE is often a disturbing and sometimes disabling condition for the 3% to 5% of the population affected by it.[21] COE represents a common pathway for several different disease states. It may be caused by allergic contact dermatitis, autoimmune disorders, chronic dermatologic conditions such as psoriasis, or chronic infection from fungi or bacteria.[4,19]

Clinical Presentation

Patients with COE present with itching of the ear, clear or mucoid otorrhea, and aural fullness. Ear pain or discomfort and hearing loss may be present if the ear canal is acutely inflamed and swollen. Many patients experience a waxing and waning course over years with intermittent exacerbations.[2] In at least half of patients, both ears are affected. At times patients may also experience AOE.[19]

Physical Examination

Physical examination findings in COE often vary depending on the cause. For example, patients with contact dermatitis may exhibit a maculopapular rash with excoriations on the skin of the conchal bowel and ear canal. Patients with chronic dermatologic conditions such as psoriasis and atopic dermatitis may show eczematous changes, hyperkeratosis, and lichenification of the ear canal epithelium. The ear canal may be weepy, erythematous, and tender as well. Seborrheic dermatitis may result in a lack of cerumen and dry, flaky, erythematous skin in the canal, with or without clear otorrhea. COE has also resulted from chronic otitis media with tympanic membrane perforation. Purulent middle-ear drainage can enter the ear canal and lead to an eczematous dermatitis. Finally, the ear canal in patients with fungal infection (otomycosis) may show fluffy, cotton-like debris. Sprouting hyphae or dots of black debris and thick otorrhea of various colors may also be observed.

Diagnosis

Diagnosis of COE is made clinically in patients with typical signs and symptoms of at least 3 months' duration.[19] Culture for bacteria and fungi is often prudent if chronic infection is suspected. Patients with possible contact dermatitis should be thoroughly questioned about the use of various agents such as neomycin, shampoos, detergents, hairsprays, and hearing-aid molds. Skin-patch testing in cases of contact dermatitis may be useful to elucidate the cause.[17] Chronic dermatologic disorders such as psoriasis should be suspected when a typical exanthem is visualized elsewhere on the skin. Finally, patients may have COE resulting from systemic autoimmune disorders already identified, such as Wegener granulomatosis and sarcoidosis.[22,23]

Treatment

Treatment of COE is aimed at identifying the underlying cause and managing accordingly. All patients should have aural toilet if needed, and be given preventive precautions as for AOE. For patients with contact dermatitis, avoidance of any potential irritants is paramount. Topical steroid therapy with medium-potency (triamcinolone 0.1% cream) and high-potency (desoximetasone 0.05% cream) agents is often effective for patients with contact dermatitis or chronic dermatologic conditions.[17,19] Cream preparations are preferred, and a small amount can be applied to the skin at the meatus twice daily. At times, higher-potency topical steroids or a short course of oral steroids may be necessary. Topical tacrolimus has also been used with success in noninfectious COE.[24]

Patients with chronic bacterial infection should be treated with topical antibiotics, as for AOE. In cases of fungal otitis externa, antifungal creams such as clotrimazole 1% may be used.[25] Acidifying topical agents are also beneficial. Gentian violet is an antifungal and drying agent that can be applied in the office.[19] It is painted on the ear canal using a home-made Q-tip (ie, a toothpick wrapped in cotton). Recalcitrant or severe cases, such as those involving *Aspergillus*, may require oral itraconazole.[4]

Complications

Patients with COE are predisposed to AOE because of the breakdown in epithelial lining resulting from excessive moisture, trauma, itching, and accumulation of debris. Fungal infection may result in perforation of tympanic membrane.[26] A major complication of COE is fibrosis of the medial canal.[27] After long-standing inflammation, a thick, fibrous scar can form at the medial end of the ear canal. The tympanic membrane may appear to be oriented laterally and have fibrotic changes, with absence of typical landmarks. Eventually a fibrotic plug may become obstructive, resulting in a blind-ending canal associated with conductive hearing loss.[19]

SUMMARY

Otitis externa is a common condition seen by primary care clinicians, who should be familiar with its diagnosis and management. AOE most often is infectious in origin, and can be easily treated with a combination of topical antibiotic and steroid preparations. Systemic antibiotics are rarely needed. COE can be more difficult to treat, but if an underlying cause can be identified this condition can often be successfully managed. In both AOE and COE, prevention is fundamental. If patients are able to avoid precipitating factors, future episodes can often be averted.

REFERENCES

1. Rowlands S, Devalia H, Smith C, et al. Otitis externa in UK general practice: a survey using the UK General Practice Research Database. Br J Gen Pract 2001; 51(468):533–8.
2. Rosenfeld RM, Brown L, Cannon CR, et al. Clinical practice guideline: acute otitis externa. Otolaryngol Head Neck Surg 2006;134(Suppl 4):S4–23.
3. Roland PS, Stroman DW. Microbiology of acute otitis externa. Laryngoscope 2002;112(7 Pt 1):1166–77.
4. Guss J, Ruckestein MJ. Infections of the external ear. In: Flint PW, Cummings CW, editors. Cummings otolaryngology head & neck surgery. 5th edition. Philadelphia: Mosby/Elsevier; 2010. p. 1944–9.
5. Russell JD, Donnelly M, McShane DP, et al. What causes acute otitis externa? J Laryngol Otol 1993;107(10):898–901.
6. Lum CL, Jeyanthi S, Prepageran N, et al. Antibacterial and antifungal properties of human cerumen. J Laryngol Otol 2009;123(4):375–8.
7. Tarazi AE, Al-Tawfiq JA, Abdi RF. Fungal malignant otitis externa: pitfalls, diagnosis, and treatment. Otol Neurotol 2012;33(5):769–73.
8. Smith IM, Keay DG, Buxton PK. Contact hypersensitivity in patients with chronic otitis externa. Clin Otolaryngol Allied Sci 1990;15(2):155–8.
9. Yariktas M, Yildirim M, Doner F, et al. Allergic contact dermatitis prevalence in patients with eczematous external otitis. Asian Pac J Allergy Immunol 2004; 22(1):7–10.
10. Jinn TH, Kim PD, Russell PT, et al. Determination of ototoxicity of common otic drops using isolated cochlear outer hair cells. Laryngoscope 2001;111(12): 2105–8.
11. Kaushik V, Malik T, Saeed SR. Interventions for acute otitis externa. Cochrane Database Syst Rev 2010;(1):Cd004740.

12. van Balen FA, Smit WM, Zuithoff NP, et al. Clinical efficacy of three common treatments in acute otitis externa in primary care: randomised controlled trial. BMJ 2003;327(7425):1201–5.
13. Mosges R, Schroder T, Baues CM, et al. Dexamethasone phosphate in antibiotic ear drops for the treatment of acute bacterial otitis externa. Curr Med Res Opin 2008;24(8):2339–47.
14. England RJ, Homer JJ, Jasser P, et al. Accuracy of patient self-medication with topical eardrops. J Laryngol Otol 2000;114(1):24–5.
15. Rubin Grandis J, Branstetter BF, Yu VL. The changing face of malignant (necrotising) external otitis: clinical, radiological, and anatomic correlations. Lancet Infect Dis 2004;4(1):34–9.
16. Schaefer P, Baugh RF. Acute otitis externa: an update. Am Fam Physician 2012; 86(11):1055–61.
17. Sood S, Strachan DR, Tsikoudas A, et al. Allergic otitis externa. Clin Otolaryngol Allied Sci 2002;27(4):233–6.
18. Collier SA, Hlavsa MC, Piercefield EW, et al. Antimicrobial and analgesic prescribing patterns for acute otitis externa, 2004-2010. Otolaryngol Head Neck Surg 2013;148(1):128–34.
19. Kesser BW. Assessment and management of chronic otitis externa. Curr Opin Otolaryngol Head Neck Surg 2011;19(5):341–7.
20. Hollis S, Evans K. Management of malignant (necrotising) otitis externa. J Laryngol Otol 2011;125(12):1212–7.
21. Ali R, Burns P, Donnelly M. Otitis externa: quality of life assessment. Ir J Med Sci 2008;177(3):221–3.
22. Illum P, Thorling K. Otological manifestations of Wegener's granulomatosis. Laryngoscope 1982;92(7 Pt 1):801–4.
23. Lang EE, el Zaruk J, Colreavy MP, et al. An unusual case of external ear inflammation caused by sarcoidosis. Ear Nose Throat J 2003;82(12):942–5.
24. Caffier PP, Harth W, Mayelzadeh B, et al. Tacrolimus: a new option in therapy-resistant chronic external otitis. Laryngoscope 2007;117(6):1046–52.
25. Vennewald I, Klemm E. Otomycosis: diagnosis and treatment. Clin Dermatol 2010;28(2):202–11.
26. Viswanatha B, Sumatha D, Vijayashree MS. Otomycosis in immunocompetent and immunocompromised patients: comparative study and literature review. Ear Nose Throat J 2012;91(3):114–21.
27. Luong A, Roland PS. Acquired external auditory canal stenosis: assessment and management. Curr Opin Otolaryngol Head Neck Surg 2005;13(5):273–6.

Acute Otitis Media

Gretchen Dickson, MD, MBA

KEYWORDS

- Acute otitis media • Otitis media with effusion • Antibiotics • Tympanostomy tube

KEY POINTS

- Acute otitis media (AOM) is a common condition seen in primary care offices, as 1 in 4 children will have at least 1 episode of AOM by age 10 years.
- AOM results from infection of fluid that has become trapped in the middle ear.
- The bacteria that most often cause AOM are *Streptococcus pneumoniae*, *Haemophilus influenzae*, and *Moraxella catarrhalis*.
- Differentiating AOM from otitis media with effusion (OME) is a critical skill for physicians, as accurate diagnosis will guide appropriate treatment of these conditions.
- Although fluid is present in the middle ear in both conditions, the fluid is not infected in OME as is seen in AOM patients.

Acute otitis media (AOM) is a common condition seen in primary care offices, as 1 in 4 children will have at least 1 episode of AOM by age 10 years.[1] AOM results from infection of fluid that has become trapped in the middle ear. The bacteria that most often cause AOM are *Streptococcus pneumoniae*, *Haemophilus influenzae*, and *Moraxella catarrhalis*. Differentiating AOM from otitis media with effusion (OME) is a critical skill for physicians, as accurate diagnosis will guide appropriate treatment of these conditions. Although fluid is present in the middle ear in both conditions, the fluid is not infected in OME as is seen in AOM patients.

EPIDEMIOLOGY

Children from a myriad of diverse demographic categories are commonly affected by AOM, although those of male gender and Native American ethnicity have been shown to be at increased risk of AOM.[2] Children who have other siblings in the home, are of low socioeconomic status, experienced premature birth, were bottle fed, have a family history of recurrent AOM, or attend out-of-home day care are also at increased risk of developing AOM.[2,3] Eliminating exposure to passive tobacco smoke, encouraging breastfeeding, and advocating for reduced pacifier use during months 7 to 12 of life may have some impact on reducing the incidence of AOM.[2] More study is needed

Department of Family and Community Medicine, University of Kansas School of Medicine-Wichita, 1010 North Kansas, Wichita, KS 67214, USA
E-mail address: gdickson@kumc.edu

Prim Care Clin Office Pract 41 (2014) 11–18
http://dx.doi.org/10.1016/j.pop.2013.10.002   **primarycare.theclinics.com**
0095-4543/14/$ – see front matter © 2014 Elsevier Inc. All rights reserved.

to clarify the impact of public health programs that optimize maternal health, encourage breastfeeding, and advocate tobacco cessation on rates of AOM.

Although a single episode of AOM may seem trivial, more than 2.2 million episodes occur annually in the United States at a cost of 4 billion dollars.[4–6] Children with recurrent episodes of AOM are most at risk for complications leading to morbidity and mortality. Early onset of a first episode may be an important marker of children most at risk to have recurrent episodes of disease.[3,7]

PREVENTION

Given the high prevalence of AOM, much research attention has focused on identifying prevention strategies. S pneumoniae, M catarrhalis, and H influenzae continue to cause most cases of AOM. Introduction of the pneumococcal vaccine has resulted in reduction of risk of up to 34% for children to develop AOM.[8,9] The impact of the 13-valent pneumococcal vaccine in current use has not yet been elucidated. Although pneumococcal vaccine certainly does not eliminate the risk of AOM for a given child, even small reductions in risk for an individual has large implications for the community regarding reductions in AOM incidence. Pneumococcal vaccine is beneficial, but children who have been fully vaccinated still contract AOM.

Widespread use of the influenza vaccine has also been shown to be effective in reducing the incidence of AOM.[10] With fewer viral illnesses, children are less likely to have inflammation and swelling of the Eustachian tube and less fluid accumulation in the middle ear. Ultimately, with less fluid accumulation and, subsequently, less bacterial colonization of the fluid, fewer ear infections occur. In one study, children who received seasonal influenza vaccine had fewer episodes of AOM, less need for antibiotics, and a shorter duration of middle-ear effusion.[10]

In addition to vaccines, other interventions designed to reduce viral upper respiratory infection or bacterial colonization of the middle ear have been studied for their ability to decrease AOM rates. Dietary supplementation has been popular, as evidence exists to suggest that deficiencies in zinc, vitamin A, vitamin D, and specific omega-3 fatty acids may result in an increased risk of AOM.[11,12] However, while specific nutritional deficiencies have been linked to increased rates of AOM, studies have demonstrated mixed evidence, at best, that supplementation for deficiencies results in a protective effect. For example, zinc has been shown to prevent AOM in malnourished children younger than 5 years, but benefit in children with normal nutritional status has not been significant enough to warrant recommendations for universal administration.[11,13,14] Moreover, supplementation for hypovitaminosis D, defined as serum levels of (OH)D of less than 30 ng/mL, has been shown to reduce the incidence of uncomplicated AOM.[12]

Probiotics have also been shown to have some benefit in decreasing the rate of AOM. Infant formulas supplemented with lactobacillus rhamnosus GG and bifidobacterium lactis Bb-12 have been shown to reduce incidence of AOM by 22% to 50% in the first 7 months of life.[15] In older children, however, the benefit is less clear. Studies have demonstrated that probiotic administration may decrease days of day care missed, but data regarding reduction in incidence rates is mixed.[11]

Xylitol, a polyol sugar alcohol found in raspberries, has been shown to be effective in preventing AOM, although most physicians who care for children are unaware of its effectiveness as a preventive agent.[16] However, to be effective xylitol must be given 5 times per day, creating a barrier to its widespread use. Beyond dietary interventions, it has been suggested that osteopathic manipulation may lead to reduction in symptoms in children with AOM, although more studies are needed to clarify any possible effect.[17]

DIAGNOSIS

Guidelines published by the American Academy of Pediatrics in 2013 acknowledge that AOM has a spectrum of presentations.[18] Diagnosis should be based on individual history and physical examination findings, with the goal of reducing overdiagnosis of AOM. A diagnosis of AOM is appropriate in children with moderate to severe bulging of the tympanic membrane, or new onset of otorrhea not attributable to acute otitis externa.[18] Similarly, children with mild bulging of the tympanic membrane and either recent onset of ear pain or intense erythema of the tympanic membrane likely have AOM.[18] Middle-ear effusion alone is not sufficient evidence of AOM.[18]

OME may be misdiagnosed and misclassified as AOM. Like AOM, OME is common, with 2.2 million episodes occurring annually at an estimated cost of $4 billion.[2,19] Often an episode of OME follows a viral upper respiratory infection, but may also occur as an episode of AOM is resolving.[2] To further complicate the diagnosis, the presence of fluid in the middle ear that occurs with OME can be colonized with bacteria and precede an episode of AOM. The major factor that distinguishes AOM and OME is that OME is not an infectious process and, as such, there should not be signs of infection such as an erythematous tympanic membrane or otalgia. Pneumatic otoscopy can be helpful in diagnosing OME.[20] Most episodes of OME will resolve spontaneously within 3 months of onset, thus watchful waiting is often the first-line treatment.[20,21] During the period of watchful waiting, antibiotics, oral glucocorticoids, intranasal glucocorticoids, antihistamines, and decongestants have not been shown to be beneficial in resolving the effusion or restoring hearing.[20] If the child is at risk of language delay because of impaired hearing or if the effusion has been present for more than 3 months, referral to an otolaryngologist for possible tympanostomy tube placement should be considered.[20] Up to 40% of children will have recurrences of OME and, depending on frequency of recurrence, these children may also benefit from tympanostomy tube placement.[21]

TREATMENT

In recent years there has been much controversy over the treatment of AOM. Following release of the 2004 guidelines developed by the American Academy of Pediatrics and the American Academy of Family Physicians that recommended more watchful waiting for AOM, several studies found that physicians were reluctant to follow these guidelines and continued to regularly prescribe antibiotics for AOM.[22,23] In 2013 updated guidelines were published by the American Academy of Pediatrics, which included new recommendations for the treatment of AOM.

ANALGESIA

AOM is associated with significant pain that may persist for up to 7 days despite antibiotic therapy.[24] A critical component of any treatment plan for AOM is determining how best to provide adequate analgesia for the patient.

Oral medications may be helpful in providing analgesia. Ibuprofen and acetaminophen have been shown to be effective in reducing AOM-related pain.[25] Narcotic medications have also been shown to be effective, although the side effects of respiratory depression and altered mental status limit the usefulness of these medications in practice.[25] Some clinicians have used antihistamines and decongestants in attempts to reduce the fluid volume in the middle ear and thus provide pain relief. However, there is no evidence that use of antihistamines or decongestants provides benefit, and a 5- to 8-fold increase in the risk of side effects is a cause for concern.[26]

Topical medications may provide adequate pain relief without systemic side effects. Procaine and phenazone have been shown to be fairly effective in reducing pain. In one study of 428 children aged 0 to 6 years, pain scores decreased significantly after using otic drops containing procaine and phenazone.[27] Benzocaine topical preparations are also an option, as use of benzocaine has been demonstrated to have minimal side effects and to provide analgesia superior to acetaminophen alone.[28]

In addition to the oral and topical medications approved by the Food and Drug Administration for pain relief in AOM, many parents have used naturopathic topical remedies. The parents of up to 46% of children aged 1 to 7 years who have recurrent episodes of AOM have administered some complementary or alternative method to their children as analgesia or treatment.[29] Some evidence exists that naturopathic drops may be equal in effectiveness to phenazone and procaine solutions.[30]

In addition to medication, tympanostomy and osteopathic manipulation have been used to alleviate pain with AOM. Tympanostomy is effective at reducing pain, but the skill required to perform this procedure limits its usefulness as an intervention in a primary care office.[2] Further study of osteopathic manipulation is also needed to determine its effectiveness, although some studies have suggested symptom reduction.[17]

ANTIBIOTIC THERAPY

Each year $2.8 billion is spent on antibiotics to treat episodes of AOM,[31] despite existing evidence that up to 78% of AOM episodes will resolve spontaneously.[32] Determining which patients to observe and which to treat with antibiotics at the time of diagnosis can be a difficult decision.

Guidelines released by the American Academy of Pediatrics in 2013 suggest that all children aged 6 months and older with evidence of AOM and otorrhea or severe symptoms such as a toxic appearance, persistent otalgia for more than 48 hours, temperature greater than 39°Celsius in the last 48 hours, or uncertain access to follow-up should be treated with antibiotics.[18] In addition, children aged 6 to 24 months who have bilateral AOM without otorrhea or severe symptoms should be treated with antibiotics.[18]

Over the last decade, treatment guidelines for AOM have included a role for observation without immediate antibiotic therapy for appropriate candidate patients. Candidates for observation include children age 6 to 24 months with unilateral AOM without otorrhea or severe symptoms or children older than 24 months with unilateral or bilateral AOM without otorrhea or severe symptoms.[18] Current guidelines on when to offer observation or antibiotic therapy are included in **Table 1**.

Table 1
Treatment options for acute otitis media (AOM)

Age of Child	AOM with Otorrhea		AOM Without Otorrhea		AOM with Severe Symptoms[a]	
	Unilateral	Bilateral	Unilateral	Bilateral	Unilateral	Bilateral
0–6 mo	Antibiotics	Antibiotics	Antibiotics	Antibiotics	Antibiotics	Antibiotics
6 mo–2 y	Antibiotics	Antibiotics	Antibiotics or observation	Antibiotics	Antibiotics	Antibiotics
>2 y	Antibiotics	Antibiotics	Antibiotics or observation	Antibiotics or observation	Antibiotics	Antibiotics

[a] Severe symptoms include: toxic-appearing child, persistent otalgia for >48 hours, temperature >39°C in past 48 hours, or uncertain access to follow-up.
Adapted from Liberthal AS, Carroll AE, Chonmaitree T, Ganiats TG, et al. The diagnosis and management of acute otitis media. Pediatrics 2013;131:e964–99

When a decision is made to use antibiotics, amoxicillin as a first line agent at a dose of 80 to 90 mg/kg/d is recommended.[2] If a child has taken amoxicillin in the prior 30 days or has conjunctivitis, high-dose amoxicillin/clavulanate (90 mg/kg/d amoxicillin and 6.4 mg/kg/d of clavulanate) is recommended.[18] If a child has a penicillin allergy, cefdinir, cefuroxime, cefpodoxime, or ceftriaxone may be used.[18]

Children with tympanic membrane perforations should be treated with oral antibiotics, whereas those with tympanostomy tubes in place should have topical ciprofloxacin/dexamethasone prescribed.[33]

A child should be reassessed in 48 to 72 hours if not improving, and treatment at that time may be changed to high-dose amoxicillin/clavulanate, ceftriaxone, or clindamycin.[18] Given the various resistance patterns of bacterial organisms, a child who fails to improve on amoxicillin should not be offered erythromycin, azithromycin, clarithromycin, or trimethoprim/sulfamethoxazole.[2] A child who continues to worsen may undergo tympanocentesis to enable culture of middle-ear fluid while continuing on an alternative treatment regimen.[18]

Duration of treatment is an important consideration. For children younger than 2 years, a 10-day course of treatment is recommended.[18] Older children may improve with a 5- to 7-day course of treatment with fewer antibiotic-related side effects.[18]

Although both the American Academy of Family Physicians and the American Academy of Pediatrics support the use of amoxicillin as a first-line, cost-effective agent for the treatment of AOM, many providers choose other medications.[23] If even 14% of the children who receive cefdinir were instead treated with amoxicillin, for example, $34 million in antibiotic costs would be saved annually.[23]

OBSERVATION

In appropriately selected patients, observation for AOM may prevent antibiotic-related side effects without significantly increasing the risk of complications from AOM. For every 100 healthy children with AOM, 80 will improve within 3 days without antibiotic therapy.[34] If all 100 children were treated with amoxicillin or ampicillin, 92 would improve although up to 10 would develop a rash and up to 10 would develop diarrhea.[34] Thus, preventing exposure to antibiotics may prevent undesirable side effects.

Many clinicians hesitate to suggest observation for AOM for fear that by withholding an antibiotic a child will develop mastoiditis or other sequelae. Although antibiotics do significantly decrease the risk of mastoiditis, 4800 children must be treated to prevent 1 case of mastoiditis.[35] Furthermore, no studies have demonstrated a resurgence of meningitis with the implementation of watchful waiting guidelines for AOM.[3]

When choosing observation as an initial management strategy, the patient must be able to return to the office or obtain antibiotics if he or she fails to improve within 48 to 72 hours of onset of AOM symptoms.[18] In fact, up to one-third of patients with AOM who choose observation may eventually need rescue antibiotics.[36]

SURGICAL OPTIONS

Children with recurrent episodes of AOM should be considered for placement of tympanostomy tubes. Referral for evaluation for tympanostomy tubes is recommended when a child has 3 or more episodes of AOM within a 6-month period or 4 episodes within a year with 1 in the preceding 6 months.[37] Age at first episode of AOM has been suggested as an important variable in considering referral for tympanostomy tubes.[37] Children who present with AOM early in life, such as before 6 months of age, may warrant a more aggressive approach to management.[37]

Surgical and anesthetic risk of tympanostomy tube placement should be compared with the benefit that tympanostomy tubes can provide in improving the quality of life and speech in children, as well as alleviation of caregiver distress and fewer recurrent AOM episodes.[18]

SUMMARY

All primary care providers who care for children will commonly care for those with AOM. Careful attention to accurate diagnosis and differentiating AOM from OME will prevent unnecessary use of antibiotics. Promoting immunization, breastfeeding, and avoidance of tobacco smoke may help to prevent AOM. Once diagnosed, determining the optimal treatment strategy, including analgesia for otalgia and appropriate use of antibiotics, is a critical task for physicians.

REFERENCES

1. Majeed A, Harris T. Acute otitis media in children. BMJ 1997;315:321–2.
2. Teele DW, Klein JO, Rosner B, et al. Epidemiology of otitis media during the first seven years of life in children in greater Boston: a prospective cohort study. J Infect Dis 1989;160(1):83–94.
3. Ladomenou F, Kafatos A, Tselentis Y, et al. Predisposing factors for acute otitis media in infancy. J Infect 2010;61(1):49–53.
4. Browning G, Rovers M, Williamson I, et al. Grommets (ventilation tubes) for hearing loss associated with otitis media with effusion in children. Cochrane Database Syst Rev 2010;(10):CD001801.
5. Trune D, Zheng Q. Mouse models for human otitis media. Brain Res 2009;1277: 90–103.
6. Ahmed S, Shapiro NL, Bhattacharyya N. Incremental health care utilization and costs for acute otitis media in children. Laryngoscope 2013. [Epub Ahead of print].
7. Pelton S, Leibovitz E. Recent advances in otitis media. Pediatr Infect Dis J 2009; 28(Suppl 10):S133–7.
8. Jansen AG, Hak E, Veenhoven RH, et al. Pneumococcal conjugate vaccines for preventing otitis media. Cochrane Database Syst Rev 2009;(2):CD001480.
9. Casey J, Adlowitz D, Pichichero M. New patterns in the otopathogens causing acute otitis media six to eight years after introduction of the pneumococcal conjugate vaccine. Pediatr Infect Dis J 2010;29(4):304–9.
10. Marchisio P, Espositio S, Bianchini S. Efficacy of injectable trivalent virosomal adjuvanted inactivated influenza vaccine in preventing acute otitis media in children with recurrent complicated or noncomplicated acute otitis media. Pediatr Infect Dis J 2009;28(10):855–9.
11. Levi JR, Brody RM, McKee-Cole K, et al. Complementary and alternative medicine for pediatric otitis media. Int J Pediatr Otorhinolaryngol 2013;77(6):926–31.
12. Marchisio P, Consonni D, Baggi E, et al. Vitamin D supplementation reduces the risk of acute otitis media in otitis-prone children. Pediatr Infect Dis J 2013;32: 1055–60.
13. Abba K, Gulani A, Sachdev H. Zinc supplements for preventing otitis media. Cochrane Database Syst Rev 2010;(2):CD006639.
14. Marchisio P, Esposito S, Bianchini S, et al. Effectiveness of a propolis and zinc solution in preventing acute otitis media in children with a history of recurrent acute otitis media. Int J Immunopathol Pharmacol 2010;23(2):567–75.

15. Rautava S, Salminen S, Isolauri E. Specific probiotics in reducing the risk of acute infections in infancy–a randomised double blind, placebo-controlled study. Br J Nutr 2009;101(11):1722–6.
16. Danhauer J, Johnson CE, Rotan SN, et al. National survey of pediatricians' opinions about and practices for acute otitis media and xylitol use. J Am Acad Audiol 2010;21(5):329–46.
17. Posadzki P, Lee MS, Ernst E. Osteopathic manipulative treatment for pediatric conditions: a systematic review. Pediatrics 2013;132:140–52.
18. Liberthal AS, Carroll AE, Chonmaitree T, et al. The diagnosis and management of acute otitis media. Pediatrics 2013;131:e.964–99.
19. Shekelle P, Takata G, Chan L. Diagnosis, natural history and late effects of otitis media with effusion. Evidence Report/Technology Assessment No. 55. Rockville (MD): Agency for Healthcare Research and Quality; 2003. p. E023 AHRQ Publication No 03.
20. American Academy of Family Physicians, American Academy of Otolaryngology-Head and Neck Surgery, American Academy of Pediatrics Subcommittee on Otitis Media with Effusion. Otitis media with effusion. Pediatrics 2004;113(5): 1412.
21. Williamson IG, Dunleavey J, Bain J, et al. The natural history of otitis media with effusion—a three-year study of the incidence and prevalence of abnormal tympanograms in four South West Hampshire infant and first schools. J Laryngol Otol 1994;108(11):930–4.
22. Vernacchio L, Vezina RM, Mitchell AA. Management of acute otitis media by primary care physicians: trends since the release of the 2004 American Academy of Pediatrics/American Academy of Family Physicians clinic practice guideline. Pediatrics 2007;120(2):281–7.
23. Coco A, Vernacchio L, Horst M, et al. Management of acute otitis media after publication of the 2004 AAP and AAFP clinical practice guideline. Pediatrics 2010;125(2):214–20.
24. Rovers MM, Glasziou P, Appelman CL, et al. Antibiotics for acute otitis media: an individual patient data meta-analysis. Lancet 2006;368(9545):1429–35.
25. Bertin L, Pons G, d'Arthis P. A randomized, double blind, multicentre controlled trial of ibuprofen versus acetaminophen and placebo for symptoms of acute otitis media in children. Fundam Clin Pharmacol 1996;10:387–92.
26. Coleman C, Moore M. Decongestants and antihistamines for acute otitis media in children. Cochrane Database Syst Rev 2008;(3):CD001727.
27. Adam D, Federspil P, Lukes M. Therapeutic properties and tolerance of procaine and phenazone containing ear drops in infants and very young children. Arzneimittelforschung 2009;59(10):504–12.
28. Hoberman A, Paradise JI, Reynolds EA, et al. Efficacy of Auralgan for treating ear pain in children with acute otitis media. Arch Pediatr Adolesc Med 1997;151:675–8.
29. Marchisio P, Bianchini S, Galeone C, et al. Use of complementary and alternative medicine in children with recurrent acute otitis media in Italy. Int J Immunopathol Pharmacol 2011;24:441–9.
30. Sarrell EM, Mandelberg A, Cohen HA. Efficacy of naturopathic extracts in the management of ear pain associated with acute otitis media. Arch Pediatr Adolesc Med 2001;155:796–9.
31. Soni A. Ear infections (otitis media) in children (0-17): use and expenditures. 2006. Statistical brief no. 228 2008 [cited 2010 November 20]; Available at: http://meps.ahrq.gov/mepsweb/data_files/publications/st228/stat228.shtml. Accessed November 6, 2013.

32. Sanders S, Glasziou PP, Del Mar C, et al. Antibiotics for acute otitis media in children. Cochrane Database Syst Rev 2004;(1):CD000219.
33. Wright D, Safranek S. Treatment of otitis media with perforated tympanic membrane. Am Fam Physician 2009;79(8):650–4.
34. Rosenfeld R, Kay D. Natural history of untreated otitis media. Laryngoscope 2003;113(10):1645–57.
35. Thompson PL, Gilbert RE, Long PF, et al. Effect of antibiotics for otitis media on mastoiditis in children: a retrospective cohort study using the United Kingdom general practice research database. Pediatrics 2009;125(2):424–30.
36. Tahtinen PA, Laine MK, Huovinen P, et al. A placebo controlled trial of antimicrobial treatment for acute otitis media. N Engl J Med 2011;364(2):116–26.
37. Higgins T, McCabe SJ, Bumpous JM, et al. Medical decision analysis: Indications for tympanostomy tubes in RAOM by age at first episode. Otolaryngol Head Neck Surg 2008;138(1):50–6.

Hearing Loss: Diagnosis and Management

John M. Lasak, MD[a,b,]*, Patrick Allen, MD[c], Tim McVay, DO[c],
Douglas Lewis, MD[c]

KEYWORDS

- Hearing loss • Otoacoustic emissions • Audiometry • Hearing aids

KEY POINTS

- It is important to identify the progression, whether unilateral or bilateral, and the presence or absence of associated tinnitus and vertigo in those presenting with hearing loss.
- A thorough physical examination of the pinna, external auditory canal, and middle ear is essential for establishing a diagnosis of hearing loss.
- Otoacoustic emissions (OAEs) test the function of the cochlear outer hair cells and are an excellent screening tool for hearing loss in the infant or young child. The external auditory canal and middle ear must be normal for reliable OAEs; therefore otoscopy must be accomplished before testing.
- The Weber and Rinne tuning fork tests can readily differentiate a conductive from sensorineural hearing loss in the office setting.
- Temporal bone computed tomography and gadolinium enhanced magnetic resonance imaging of the brain and internal auditory canal are the imaging modalities of choice for hearing loss.

INTRODUCTION

Hearing loss may affect all age groups from the newborn to the elderly, impacting speech and language development in children and causing social and vocational problems for adults. Hearing loss can arise from anywhere in the auditory circuit including the external auditory canal (EAC), sound conduction mechanism, cochlea, cochlear nerve, and central auditory pathways. Rehabilitation options exist for all types of hearing loss, regardless of cause or location within the auditory system. Awareness of symptoms, signs, and rehabilitative measures aids primary care physicians in early identification and treatment of hearing loss.

[a] Departments of Surgery and Pediatrics, University of Kansas School of Medicine-Wichita, Wichita, KS, USA; [b] The Wichita Ear Clinic, 9350 East Central Avenue, Wichita, KS 67206, USA; [c] Department of Family and Community Medicine, The University of Kansas School of Medicine-Wichita, 1010 North Kansas, Wichita, KS 67214, USA
* Corresponding author. The Wichita Ear Clinic, 9350 East Central Avenue, Wichita, KS 67206.
E-mail address: Jlasak1@cox.net

Prim Care Clin Office Pract 41 (2014) 19–31
http://dx.doi.org/10.1016/j.pop.2013.10.003
0095-4543/14/$ – see front matter © 2014 Elsevier Inc. All rights reserved.

EPIDEMIOLOGY

The incidence of infant hearing loss is estimated at 4 to 60 per 1000 neonates.[1] Approximately 3% of white children and adolescents experience hearing loss with estimates of hearing loss being higher among some minorities, and children from lower socioeconomic backgrounds.[2] Childhood hearing loss is often identified when a parent reports that their infant or child does not respond to voice, when speech or language delay is present, or when school performance is poor. Caregiver concern for hearing loss should prompt a physician to investigate further. Additional risk factors for hearing loss that may prompt screening are shown in **Box 1**.[1,3,4] The significant educational and social ramifications of hearing loss in children have prompted the United States Preventive Services Task Force to recommend newborn hearing screening for all neonates.[5] Approximately 95% of newborn infants in the United States are screened for hearing loss before hospital discharge.[4]

The prevalence of hearing loss in adults increases with age. Adult hearing loss often presents through family complaints to the physician or the affected becoming isolated and withdrawn in social situations prompting the family to seek care. It is estimated that 28 million adults in the United States have some degree of hearing impairment.[6] A 5-year study of 2837 adult individuals estimated the prevalence of hearing loss by age group in the United States as follows:

- Ages 21 to 34: 2.9%
- Ages 35 to 44: 6.4%
- Ages 44 to 54: 10.9%
- Ages 55 to 64: 25.1%
- Ages 65 to 84: 42.7%[7]

CLINICAL PRESENTATION

For patients presenting with hearing loss, it is important to identify the progression of loss, whether unilateral or bilateral in nature, and the presence or absence of associated tinnitus and vertigo. Noise exposure, use of ototoxic medications, illicit drug use, and medical conditions, such as diabetes, atherosclerosis, and kidney disease, are also important to note during the history. Furthermore, history of chronic otologic infections or otologic surgery should be noted. In children, intrauterine and neonatal risk factors should be identified.

DIAGNOSIS
Physical Examination

A thorough physical examination with attention to the anatomic survey of the ear is critical for establishing a diagnosis of hearing loss.[8] Obstruction of the EAC with cerumen, inflammation (otitis externa), or a foreign body may produce a conductive hearing loss. EAC atresia (with or without microtia) also causes a conductive loss with the degree of hearing loss being proportional to the severity of atresia. Findings consistent with clinical syndromes are also important to note. Craniofacial anomalies may have middle and inner ear abnormalities and associated conductive, mixed, or sensorineural loss.[9] Syndromic hearing loss, such as occurs with Treacher-Collins syndrome, Crouzon disease, or Robin sequence, accounts for 15% to 30% of hereditary etiologies.[10]

Otoscopy of the tympanic membrane (TM) to ascertain integrity, translucency, and the presence or absence of middle ear disease is a key component of the physical examination for hearing loss. Use of pneumatic otoscopy can enable a clinician to

Box 1
Risk factors for early childhood hearing loss

Caregiver concerns regarding hearing

Family history of permanent childhood hearing loss

Neonatal intensive care stay of more than 5 days

In utero infections including

- Cytomegalovirus
- Herpes
- Rubella
- Syphilis
- Toxoplasmosis

In utero exposure to

- Maternal diabetes
- Maternal drug or alcohol use

Limited prenatal care

Multiple births

Neonatal exposure to

- Extracorporeal membrane oxygenation
- Assisted ventilation
- Otoxic medications (gentamycin, tobramycin)
- Loop diuretics
- Hyperbilirubinemia requiring exchange transfusion
- Meconium aspiration

Physical examination findings including

- Anomalies of the pinna
- Anomalies of the ear canal
- Ear tags
- Ear pits
- Anomalies of the temporal bone

Evidence of or family history of inherited syndromes including

- Neurofibromatosis Type II
- Osteopetrosis
- Usher syndrome
- Waardenburg syndrome
- Alport syndrome
- Pendred syndrome
- Jervell syndrome
- Lange-Nielsen syndrome

Neurodegenerative disorders such as

- Hunter syndrome

- Friedreich ataxia

- Charcot-Marie-Tooth syndrome

Culture-positive, postnatal infections associated with sensorineural hearing loss

Retrolental fibrous dysplasia

Data from Kountakis SE, Skoulas I, Phillips D, et al. Risk factors for hearing loss in neonates: a prospective study. Am J Otol 2002;23(3):133–7; and Joint Committee on Infant Hearing. Year 2007 position statement: principles and guidelines for early hearing detection and intervention programs. Pediatrics 2007;120(4):898–921.

identify a nonmobile TM related to middle ear effusion, tympanosclerosis, cholesteatoma, or a middle ear mass. Hypermobility of the TM, however, indicates a disruption of the ossicular chain. A retracted TM that only moves with negative pressure indicates eustachian tube dysfunction.[8]

The Weber and Rinne tests are screening examinations that can assist in differentiating between conductive and sensorineural deficits.[11] Conductive losses, especially when unilateral, suggest external or middle ear disease. Sensorineural hearing losses, especially when unilateral, may suggest a Meniere's disease or an acoustic neuroma.

The Weber test can help to determine type of hearing loss (sensorineural vs conductive) in a patient with asymmetric hear loss. The Weber test is performed by pressing the handle of a 512 Hz vibrating tuning fork to the midline of the forehead, bridge of the nose, or upper dentition. The patient reports in which ear sound is loudest. If sound is heard equally in both ears, hearing is either normal or hearing loss is symmetric. When sound is louder in the "good" ear, sensorineural hearing loss is suspected in the poorer-hearing ear. In contrast, if sound is louder in the poorer-hearing ear a conductive loss is suspected.

The Rinne test is performed with a 512-Hz, vibrating tuning fork placed on the mastoid bone. A patient is asked to report when they no longer hear sound with the fork on the mastoid bone. When sound is no longer heard, the tuning fork is moved to outside of the ear on the same side. A positive, or normal, Rinne test occurs when the sound by air conduction is louder than sound by bone conduction. Conversely, a "negative" Rinne test occurs when the patient reports that they cannot hear any sound when the tuning fork is moved from the mastoid bone to outside of the EAC. In a negative Rinne test, bone conduction through the mastoid process is louder than air conduction of sound.

Combining the results of Weber and Rinne testing is especially valuable. **Table 1** describes the diagnostic implications of common findings on Weber and Rinne testing. Some children as young as 3 can give reliable tuning fork tests.

In the absence of a simple, correctable cause diagnosed by physical examination alone, all cases of progressive conductive and sensorineural hearing loss should be referred to an otologist or otolaryngologist for additional workup including audiometry and imaging.[12]

Imaging

To determine the cause of hearing loss, temporal bone computed tomography and gadolinium-enhanced magnetic resonance imaging of the brain and internal auditory canal are the imaging modalities of choice.[9] Temporal bone computed tomography may be used to confirm structural abnormalities, such as atresia, chronic otitis media, or cholesteatoma. Furthermore, all children with sensorineural hearing loss require a temporal bone computed tomography to assess for enlarged vestibular aqueduct

Table 1
The Weber and Rinne 512 Hz tuning for tests

Hearing Status	Tuning Fork Results
Normal or symmetric bilateral SNHL	Weber: midline (or equal both ears) Rinne right ear: AC>BC Rinne left ear: AC>BC
Symmetric CHL	Weber: midline (or equal both ears) Rinne right ear: BC>AC Rinne left ear: BC>AC
Right SNHL	Weber: lateralizes left Rinne right ear: AC>BC Rinne left ear: AC>BC
Left SNHL	Weber: lateralizes right Rinne right ear: AC>BC Rinne left ear: AC>BC
Right CHL	Weber: lateralizes right Rinne right ear: BC>AC Rinne left ear AC>BC
Left CHL	Weber: lateralizes left Rinne right ear: AC>BC Rinne left ear: BC>AC

Abbreviations: AC, air conduction; BC, bone conduction; CHL, conductive hearing loss; SNHL, sensorineural hearing loss; >, greater.

syndrome and other congenital cochlear and vestibular anomalies. Diagnosis of enlarged vestibular aqueduct syndrome offers important prognostic information because even minor head trauma, such as encountered in contact sports, may cause hearing to deteriorate.[13] Retrochochlear causes, such as acoustic neuroma or cochlear nerve agenesis, are identified with gadolinium-enhanced magnetic resonance imaging.[9,14]

Audiometric Evaluation

Once hearing loss is suspected, the degree of loss needs to be quantified. Different modalities are used to determine hearing in infants, children, and adults. The audiologic tests available are provided in **Box 2**.

Box 2
Common audiology tests

Tympanometry

Otoacoustic emissions

Auditory brainstem response testing

Behavioral audiometry

Speech reception threshold

Conventional air and bone audiometry

Speech discrimination score (word discrimination)

Infants and young children may not be able to actively participate during auditory testing. Therefore, passive techniques, such as tympanometry, otoacoustic emissions (OAEs), and auditory brainstem response (ABR) testing, are used. Tympanometry determines compliance of the TM and is useful for identifying middle ear effusions and perforations.

OAEs test the function of the cochlear outer hair cells and are an excellent screening tool for hearing loss in the infant or child.[15] The EAC and middle ear must be normal for reliable OAE testing; therefore, otoscopy must be accomplished before testing. Present OAEs indicate normal hearing (with the exception of auditory neuropathy), whereas their absence suggests a loss of 30 dB or greater. In auditory neuropathy the affected individual has normal OAEs; however, transmission of the signal through the auditory pathways is impaired producing an abnormal ABR test.

If auditory neuropathy is suspected or an individual fails screening testing with OAEs, then ABR testing should be performed. The ABR test delivers a series of clicks to the auditory circuit and may be accomplished in a sleeping or sedated infant. The diagnostic ABR can determine air and bone thresholds and can yield information throughout the speech frequencies providing enough data to fit the child with amplification.[16]

Behavioral, or play audiometry, may be used for infants and young children and also can provide reliable hearing thresholds adequate for aiding. During behavioral audiometry the audiologist may train the child to look toward something of interest, such as a puppet, when a sound is presented. A conditioned response to sound is created enabling the audiologist to determine the child's hearing threshold.

Conventional air and bone conduction audiometry is used in the adult patient. The speech reception threshold determines the minimum hearing level for speech in decibels. Conventional audiometry can readily differentiate sensory, conductive, and mixed types of hearing loss. Word discrimination testing is used to determine the patient's ability to discriminate a series of words. A list of words is presented at 40 dB above their speech reception threshold and they are asked to repeat the words. A word discrimination of 90% or better is considered normal. Passive tests, such as OAE and ABR, may be used in the mentally challenged adult to determine hearing thresholds.

ETIOLOGY
Embryonic Developmental Anomalies

External ear anomalies often manifest as microtia, anotia, or EAC atresia, are often associated with other craniofacial syndromes, and generally result in a CHL.[17] Inner ear anomalies, on the other hand, occur during temporal bone embryonic development, can be associated with genetic syndromes or craniofacial anomalis, and may result in conductive, sensorineural, or mixed hearing loss. Inner ear abnormalities are classified into four major divisions: (1) Michel, (2) Mondini, (3) Scheibe, and (4) Alexander.[17] The degree of hearing loss severity varies widely among patients.

Genetic Causes of Hearing Loss

Genetic anomalies that affect hearing occur in 1-2 per 1000 newborns.[18–21] Both syndromic (associated with other phenotypic anomalies) and nonsyndromic inheritence patterns exist; with non syndromic accounting for 70% of cases.[10,18–21] Hearing loss resulting from genetic causes can be sensorineural, conductive, or mixed. More than 80 loci have been linked to nonsyndromic recessive inheritance, but mutations in the GJB2 gene on chromosome 13, which encodes for the connexin 26 protein, are responsible for nearly half of all cases.[18] Nonsyndromic autosomal-dominant patterns account for 10% to 15% of cases.[18,19] Additionally, some X-linked, nonsyndromic disorders, such as mucopolysccharidosis and Alport syndrome, may have a component of hearing loss.[19]

An autosomal-dominant inheritance pattern is noted with syndromic hearing loss associated with Waardenburg, neurofibromatosis II, and brachio-oto-renal syndromes.[10] Autosomal-recessive inherited syndromes leading to hearing loss include Ushers, Pendred, and Jervell and Lange-Nilesen.[10]

Infectious

Acute otitis media (AOM) and otitis media with effusion (OME) are the most common causes of conductive hearing loss in children.[22] Fluid accumulated in the middle ear prevents normal TM vibration resulting in hearing loss.[23] The prevention, treatment, and sequelae of unresolved AOM are discussed elsewhere in this issue (Dickson, acute otitis media).

Cholesteatoma is a growth of desquamated epithelium that forms within a retraction pocket as a result of eustachian tube dysfunction, TM trauma, and inflammation. Cholesteatoma can also be primarily acquired (congenital) rather than secondarily associated with a TM perforation or eustachian tube dysfunction.[24] Cholesteatoma may expand into the middle ear and mastoid spaces with resultant chronic otorrhea, hearing loss, and local destruction.[25] The sequelae of cholesteatoma may include hearing loss, vestibular symptoms, facial nerve paralysis, subperiosteal abscess, meningitis, sepsis, lateral sinus thrombosis, brain abscess, and even death.

Hearing loss may also result from maternal infections that a child is exposed to during the perinatal period. Insult to the developing cochlea can occur with hepatitis, rubella, toxoplasmosis, HIV, syphilis, and cytomegalovirus. Cytomegalovirus has shown a 10-fold prevalence increase in congenital infection in children with hearing loss.[23,26]

Noise Exposure

Noise exposure compounded over time induces hearing loss by direct mechanical damage of cochlear structures and metabolic overload by nitric oxide and oxygen free radical damage to cochlear hair cells. The US Occupational Safety and Health Administration noise exposure guidelines require ear protection when a time-weighted average exposure of 85 dB is reached.[27] The noise of a typical power lawn mower is 90 dB. Additionally, short blasts of noise at 120 to 155 dB may cause pain and result in severe sensorineural damage.[28] Hearing protection and avoidance of noise exposure can prevent noise-induced hearing loss.

Otosclerosis

Otosclerosis is the leading cause of hearing loss in adults who do not have a history of middle ear effusion or otitis media.[29] Progressive conductive or mixed hearing loss occurs as the stapes footplate becomes impeded from normal movement in the oval window as a result of bony deposition at the stapes footplate.[8] The loss may be treated with amplification or stapedectomy.

Trauma

Conductive hearing loss from TM trauma is common and often results from a penetrating foreign body. Small perforations in the anteroinferior portion of the TM cause minimal deficit, but larger perforations in other regions can cause significant hearing loss.[8] Ossicular disruption with conductive or mixed loss must always be considered with penetrating injuries.

Large and sudden changes in ambient air pressure (sky diving, scuba diving, air bag deployment, and boxing) without equilibration by the eustachian tube can result in barotrauma to the middle or inner ear. Occasionally, even gradual pressure changes (mountain climbing, airplane travel) cause damage when an upper respiratory infection or eustachian tube dysfunction is present.[25] Injury patterns include serous effusion, hemotympanum, perforation, and structural damage with perilymph fistula formation.[30] Hearing loss, tinnitus, pressure, pain, and vertigo are common complaints.[31]

Pressure changes through blast trauma (explosions, hydraulic) can result in sensorineural losses from concussive forces on the inner ear, whereas shearing forces are capable of damaging the organ of Corti and temporal bone.

Ototoxicity

A variety of medications may have ototoxic side effects. Permanent sensorineural hearing loss has been associated with exposure to antibiotics (aminoglycosides, erythromycin, tetracycline, and vancomycin), chemotherapy (cisplatin and 5-fluorouracil), heavy metals (lead, mercury, cadmium, and arsenic), illicit drugs (cocaine), and phsophodiesterase-5 inhibitors.[14,32] Given the risk of permanent hearing loss, neomycin-containing eardrops should not be used if a TM perforation or myringotomy tube is present.[33] Sensorineural loss from high-dose (6–8 g/day) aspirin is reversible on cessation of the medication.

Acoustic Neuroma

Acoustic neuroma are typically unilateral, Schwann cell–derived tumors that occur on the vestibular portion of the eighth cranial nerve. Patients may present with symptoms arising from cranial nerve involvement, tumor growth, and brainstem compression.[34] Additionally, 95% of patients experience hearing loss, whereas 63% describe tinnitus.[35]

Autoimmune

Sensorineural hearing loss may be the primary manifestation of autoimmune disease. Hearing loss has been commonly described in such conditions as Wegener granulomatosis, Cogan syndrome, rheumatoid arthritis, lupus, or relapsing polychondritis. Autoimmune-related hearing loss tends to fluctuate over time, is usually bilateral, and often responds to steroid therapy.[36,37]

Central Auditory Processing Disorder

Central auditory processing disorder (CAPD) results from dysfunction in the central auditory portion of the cerebral cortex leading to deficit in the analysis or interpretation of auditory information. In children, CAPD should be considered if a child seems to hear, but not comprehend sound. Risk factors include hyperbilirubinemia in the neonatal period, birth asphyxia, in utero infections, and head trauma.[23] Adults may develop CAPD as a consequence of neurodegenerative disorders or cerebrovascular accident. Standard audiology testing and OAEs may be normal in CAPD, although ABR and psychoacoustic testing may show deficits leading to diagnosis.[33]

Presbycusis

Age-related hearing loss is hallmarked by a gradually progressive, symmetric, high-frequency loss. Patients with presbycusis often express concern that they are unable to understand speech, particularly in noisy environments, and often experience tinnitus. The US Preventive Services Task Force has determined that there is insufficient evidence to recommend for or against screening asymptomatic adults older than age 50.[38]

Meniere Disease

Meniere disease affects both hearing and balance. It is believed to result from an excess of inner ear fluid (endolymphatic hydrops). Patients experience fluctuating symptoms of hearing loss, tinnitus, ear fullness, and rotary vertigo with episodes lasting twenty minutes to hours.[39]

TREATMENT

The treatment of hearing loss depends on the type of loss and cause. Medical, surgical, and amplification are the three treatment modalities. Medical therapy in the form of oral and ototopical antibiotics and steroids are used for infectious and systemic etiologies.

The surgical treatment of hearing loss falls into reparative procedures as a result of infectious or traumatic etiologies, and restorative procedure to rehabilitate hearing loss that cannot be treated with conventional amplification (congenital aural atresia, profound unilateral or bilateral loss). Infectious processes, such as chronic otitis media with effusion and chronic otitis media with or without cholesteatoma, may be surgically treated with myringotomy with tubes and tympanomastoid surgery, respectfully. Tympanoplasty can be used to repair a perforated drum and restore a conductive loss. Otosclerosis, infectious, congenital, or traumatic etiologies may cause ossicular fixation or discontinuity, and a stapedectomy or ossiculoplasty may restore the sound conduction mechanism. Candidates with congenital aural atresia may undergo an atresia repair to create an EAC, TM, and ossicular chain, thereby restoring air conduction hearing.

The bone-anchored hearing aid (BAHA) is a device that can be used to restore a conductive loss that cannot be treated with conventional amplification or unilateral profound hearing loss. The BAHA is placed during a short outpatient procedure, where a titanium abutment is placed in the retroauricular region and a sound processor is attached to it. The sound then conducts through the abutment and skull base to the functioning cochlea. This novel device can even be placed on the deaf side in those with unilateral deafness thus enabling bone conduction to the normal contralateral cochlea and improved speech perception in noise.[40]

Cochlear implants are sophisticated devices used to rehabilitate those with bilateral profound sensory hearing loss. The cochlear implant bypasses a nonfunctional cochlea and directly stimulates the cochlear nerve. This device is approved for adults and children 1 year or older.[41] Children identified with profound hearing loss and those with severe to profound loss that do not reach speech and communication milestones with amplification should be implanted as soon as possible.[42–44] Bilateral cochlear implantation improves speech and language acquisition in children and is becoming the standard of care worldwide.[41] Many children implanted early are able to enter mainstream school and develop normal speech.[41] Implanted adult communication gains often enable return to the workforce, telephone use, and for some the ability to enjoy music again.

Some patients with profound hearing loss may not be cochlear implant candidates because of the absence of functional cochlear nerves. This is most frequently encountered in patients with neurofibromatosis type 2, congenital cochlear nerve aplasia, and skull base bony dysplasia. The auditory brainstem implant may be used in patients without an intact cochlear nerve. An auditory brainstem implant directly stimulates the cochlear nucleus and most patients have improved sound awareness and enhanced lipreading.[45]

ASSISTIVE LISTENING DEVICES AND AMPLIFICATION

Amplification and assistive listening devices are the mainstay for treating hearing loss. By carefully matching device recommendations to patient needs and preferences, physicians can improve social function, communication, and emotional well-being of patients.[46]

Assistive listening devices may provide amplification or may substitute visual and tactile signals for sounds. Internet telephony, or Voice over Internet Protocol, is able to transmit more of the natural human speech frequency range than a traditional telephone, and can improve comprehension significantly.[47] Such solutions should be individualized to meet patient needs and patient preferences to optimize patient use of devices.[48]

Although hearing loss is common, particularly in older adults, hearing aid use is limited. As many as 30% of adults with hearing aids do not use them on a consistent basis and up to 75% of adults who could benefit from amplification never even acquire hearing aids.[46,49] Hearing aid ownership and use cannot be predicted by age, education level, functional impairment, or medication use.[50] Patient confidence that communication will improve is the biggest motivator for acquiring and using hearing aids.[51] When compared with unassisted hearing-impaired adults, hearing aid users have less depression, less social isolation, increased cognitive function, and improved relationships.[52,53] Barriers to obtaining and using hearing aids include concerns related to convenience of use, cost, social norms, negative stereotypes, and reported experience of others.[48] Additional barriers to regular use may include limits on manual dexterity necessary to insert, remove, and clean the device; uncomfortable fit; or difficulty adapting to sound quality when amplified through the hearing aid.[54] Parents of hearing-impaired children may be subject to denial, and should be educated on the linguistic and social gains that amplification can afford their children.[55]

The type of hearing aid selected by an individual is largely determined by patient perceptions of appearance, ease of use, and physician recommendation.[56] Behind-the-ear, in-the-ear, in-the-canal, and completely in-the-canal hearing aids differ on size, placement in or outside of the ear, and the degree to which they amplify sound.[57] Improvements in fit and technology have allowed hearing aids to become smaller, more comfortable, and capable of producing more natural sound with less extraneous noise.[57]

The Lyric (InSound Medical, Newark, CA, USA) is a new completely in-the-canal model that is the smallest and least visible external hearing device currently available. It is inserted by a professional in the office and remains in the meatus for as long as 4 months. Because it does not require battery changes or daily insertion, the low maintenance requirement for Lyric is attractive to many individuals. Although users can shower, full water immersion is not recommended.

In addition to hearing aids worn in the affected ear to amplify sound, contralateral routing of signal (CROS) aids can be used for unilateral hearing loss. These devices are intended to deliver sound from the deaf side to the good ear. A transmitter placed on deaf side transfers sound wirelessly to the hearing ear. A newer technology, the TransEar (Ear Technology Corporation, Johnson City, TN, USA), is a hearing aid with a deep-seated ear mold that couples to the bony EAC enabling bone conduction through the skull base to the contralateral cochlea.[58] This device acts similarly to the

BAHA; however, the deep-seated ear mold may at times be uncomfortable. The BiCROS aid can be used in a person with unilateral deafness that also has some degree of hearing loss in the good ear. The BiCROS aid uses the same technology as the CROS; however, the receiving ear also has an amplifier to improve its ability to hear. Bone aids can be used in those who cannot use a traditional aid, such as in an infant with atresia. The aid couples to the mastoid segment and enables bone conduction to the cochlea located within the osseous skull base.

SUMMARY

The primary care physician will undoubtedly encounter hearing loss in patients of all ages during their practice, and may be presented with the challenge of identifying and coordinating a treatment plan. Management in the form of medical, surgical, and amplification can have a dramatic impact on function and quality of life for the hearing impaired. Consultation with an otologist, orotolarygologist, and an audiologist enables early and appropriate intervention in those patients who need additional rehabilitation.

REFERENCES

1. Northern JL, Hayes D. Universal screening for infant hearing impairments: necessary, beneficial and justifiable. Audiol Today 1994;6(3):10–3.
2. Haddad J. Hearing loss. In: Kliegman RM, Stanton BF, Schor NF, et al, editors. Nelson textbook of pediatrics. 19th edition. Atlanta (GA): Elsevier/Saunders; 2011. p. 2188–93.
3. Kountakis SE, Skoulas I, Phillips D, et al. Risk factors for hearing loss in neonates: a prospective study. Am J Otol 2002;23(3):133–7.
4. Joint Committee on Infant Hearing. Year 2007 position statement: principles and guidelines for early hearing detection and intervention programs. Pediatrics 2007;120(4):898–921.
5. USPSTF. Universal screening for hearing loss in newborns. Available at: http://www.uspreventiveservicestaskforce.org/. Accessed March 2013.
6. Van Vliet D. The current status of hearing care: can we change the status quo? J Am Acad Audiol 2005;16(7):410–8.
7. Nash SD, Cruickshanks KJ, Klein R, et al. The 5-year incidence and progression of hearing loss: the epidemiology of hearing loss study. Arch Otolaryngol Head Neck Surg 2011;137(5):432.
8. Isaacson JE, Vora NM. Differential diagnosis and treatment of hearing loss. Am Fam Physician 2003;68:1125–32.
9. St Martin MB, Hirsch BE. Imaging of hearing loss. Otolaryngol Clin North Am 2008;41:157–78.
10. Gurtler N, Lalwani AK. Etiology of syndromic and nonsymdromic sensorineural hearing loss. Otolaryngol Clin North Am 2002;35:891–908.
11. Behn A, Westerberg BD, Zhang H, et al. Accuracy of the Weber and Rinne tuning fork tests in evaluation of children with otitis media with effusion. J Otolaryngol 2007;36(4):197–202.
12. Rauch SD. Idiopathic sudden sensorineural hearing loss. N Engl J Med 2008; 359:833–40.
13. Lasak JM, Welling DB. The enlarged vestibular aqueduct syndrome. Curr Opin Otolaryngol Head Neck Surg 2000;8(5):380–3.
14. Chau JK, Cho JJ, Dieter KF. Evidence-based practice: management of adult sensorineural hearing loss. Otolaryngol Clin North Am 2012;45:941–58.

15. Bhatia P, Mintz S, Hecht BF, et al. Early identification of young children with hearing loss in federally qualified health centers. J Dev Behav Pediatr 2013;34:15–21.
16. Nelson HD, Bougastos C, Nygren P. Universal newborn hearing screening: systematic review to update the 2001 U.S. Preventive services Task Force Recommendation. Rockville (MD): Agency for Healthcare Research and Quality (US); 2008. Report No. 08-05117-EF-1. Available at: US Preventive Services Task Force Evidence Syntheses, formerly Systematic Evidence reviews.
17. Rodriguez K, Shah RK, Kenna M. Anomalies of the middle and inner ear. Otolaryngol Clin North Am 2007;40:81–96.
18. Thomas MA, Der Kaloustin VM, Tewfik TL. Connexin mutation testing of children with nonsyndromic, autosomal recessive sensorineural hearing loss. J Otolaryngol 2004;33(3):189–92.
19. Willems PJ. Genetic causes of hearing loss. N Engl J Med 2000;342:1101–9.
20. Cohen M, Phillips JA. Genetic approach to evaluation of hearing loss. Otolaryngol Clin North Am 2012;45:25–39.
21. Morton NE. Genetic epidemiology of hearing impairment. Ann N Y Acad Sci 1991;630:16–31.
22. Bluestone CD, Klein JO. Otitis media, atelectasis, and eustachian tube dysfunction. In: Bluestone CD, Stool SE, Scheetz MD, editors. Pediatric otolaryngology. 2nd edition. Philadelphia: Saunders; 1990. p. 320–486.
23. Roizen NJ. Etiology of hearing loss in children: nongenetic causes. Pediatr Clin North Am 1999;46:49–64.
24. Semaan MT, Megerian CA. The pathophysiology of cholesteatoma. Otolaryngol Clin North Am 2006;39:1143–59.
25. Ely JW, Hansen MR, Clark EC. Diagnosis of ear pain. Am Fam Physician 2008; 77(5):621–8.
26. Misono S, Kathleen CY, Weiss NS, et al. Congenital cytomegalovirus infection in pediatric hearing loss. Arch Otolaryngol Head Neck Surg 2011;137:47–53.
27. Recommendations for a noise standard. In: Occupational noise exposure: NIOSH Publication Number 98–126/CDC/NIOSH.
28. Rabinowitz PM. Noise-induced hearing loss. Am Fam Physician 2000;61(9): 2749–56.
29. Emmett JR. Physical examination and clinical evaluation of the patient with otosclerosis. Otolaryngol Clin North Am 1993;26:353–7.
30. Lasak JM, VanEss M, Kryzer TC, et al. Middle ear injury through the external auditory canal: a review of 44 cases. Ear Nose Throat J 2006;85(11):724–8.
31. Lynch JH, Bove AA. Diving medicine: a review of current evidence. J Am Board Fam Med 2009;22:399–407.
32. Shargorodsky J, Curhan SG, Henderson E, et al. Heavy metals exposure and hearing loss in US adolescents. Arch Otolaryngol Head Neck Surg 2011;137:1183–9.
33. Kral A, O'Donoghue GM. Profound deafness in childhood. N Engl J Med 2010; 363:1438–50.
34. Welling DB, Lasak JM. Vestibular schwannoma. In: Glasscock ME, Gulya AJ, editors. Glasscock-shambaugh surgery of the ear. 5th edition. Ontario (Canada): BC Decker; 2002. p. 641–80.
35. Matttheis C, Samii M. Management of 1000 vestibular schwannomas (acoustic neuromas): clinical presentation. Neurosurgery 1997;40(1):1–9.
36. Ruckenstein MJ. Autoimmune inner ear disease. Curr Opin Otolaryngol Head Neck Surg 2004;12(5):426–30.
37. Lasak JM, Sataloff RT, Hawkshaw, et al. Autoimmune inner ear disease: steroid and cytotoxic drug therapy. Ear Nose Throat J 2001;80(11):808–22.

38. Moyer VA, on behalf of the U.S. Preventive Services Task Force. Screening for hearing loss in older adults: U.S. Preventive Services Task Force recommendation statement. Ann Intern Med 2012;157(9):655–61.
39. Sajjadi H, Paparella MM. Meniere's disease. Lancet 2008;372:406–14.
40. Nicolas S, Mohamed A, Yoann P, et al. Long-term benefit and sound localization in patients with single-sided deafness rehabilitated with an osseointegrated bone-conduction device. Otol Neurotol 2013;34(1):111–4.
41. Ramsden JD, Gordon K, Aschendorff A, et al. European bilateral pediatric cochlear implant forum consensus statement. Otol Neurotol 2012;33(4):561–5.
42. Geers AE, Nicholas JG. Enduring advantages of early cochlear implantation for spoken language development. J Speech Lang Hear Res 2013;56(2):643–55.
43. Clark JH, Wang NY, Riley AW, et al. Timing of cochlear implantation and parents global rating of children's health and development. Otol Neurotol 2012;33: 545–52.
44. Fulcher A, Purcell AA, Baker E, et al. Listen up: children with early identified hearing loss achieve age-appropriate speech/language outcomes by 3 years of age. Int J Pediatr Otorhinolaryngol 2012;76(12):1785–94.
45. Colletti L, Shannon R, Collettis V. Auditory brainstem implants for neurofibromatosis type 2. Curr Opin Otolaryngol Head Neck Surg 2012;20(5):353–7.
46. Mulrow CD, Aguilar C, Endicott JE, et al. Quality-of-life changes and hearing impairment. A randomized trial. Ann Intern Med 1990;113(3):188–94.
47. Mantokoudis G, Dubach P, Pfiffner F, et al. Speech perception benefits of internet versus conventional telephony for hearing impaired individuals. J Med Internet Res 2012;14(4):e102.
48. Pacal JT, Yueh B. Hearing deficits in the older patient: "I didn't notice anything." JAMA 2012;307(11):1185–94.
49. Popelka MM, Cruickshanks KJ, Wiley TL, et al. Low prevalence of hearing aid use among older adults with hearing loss: the Epidemiology of Hearing Loss Study. J Am Geriatr Soc 1998;46(9):1075–8.
50. Kochkin S. MarkeTrak IV: what is the viable market for hearing aids? Hear J 1997;50(1):31–9.
51. Gussekloo J, de Bont LE, von Faber M, et al. Auditory rehabilitation of older people from the general population—the Leiden 85-plus study. Br J Gen Pract 2003; 53(492):536–40.
52. Kochkin S, Rogin CM. Quantifying the obvious: the impact of hearing aids on quality of life. Hear Rev 2000;7(1):8–34.
53. Hutchison B, Covan EK, Bogus JC. Presbycusis. Part 1: can you hear the music of life? Care Manag J 2012;13(3):148–72.
54. Yueh B, Souza PE, McDowell JA, et al. Randomized trial of amplification strategies. Arch Otolaryngol Head Neck Surg 2001;127(10):1197–204.
55. Munoz K, Blaiser K, Barwick K. Parent hearing aid experiences in the United States. J Am Acad Audiol 2013;24(1):5–16.
56. Yueh B, Shapiro N, MacLean CH, et al. Screening and management of adult hearing loss in primary care: scientific review. JAMA 2003;289(15):1976–85.
57. Hearing Aids. National Institute on Deafness and Other Communication Disorders. Available at: http://www.nidcd.nih.gov/health/hearing/pages/hearingaid.aspx. Accessed April 15, 2013.
58. Battista RA, Nullens K, Weiet RM, et al. Sound localization in unilateral deafness with the BAHA or TransEar device. JAMA Otolaryngol Head Neck Surg 2013; 139(1):64–70.

Rhinitis

Sheryl Beard, MD

KEYWORDS

- Rhinitis • Allergy • Antihistamine • Nasal congestion

KEY POINTS

- Seasonal allergic rhinitis is commonly caused by a variety of pollen allergens. Perennial allergic rhinitis is mainly caused by dust mites and animal dander. Occupational rhinitis results from airborne particles in the workplace and is a response to allergic and nonallergic mechanisms.
- Mild disease can usually be managed with avoidance measures alone. Allergen removal can also improve the severity of allergic rhinitis and can reduce the need for medications. Pollen, dust mites, animals, insect proteins, and fungi are the most prominent allergic triggers. Environmental control may take weeks to months to produce full beneficial effects, and complete avoidance of allergen is usually not feasible or practical.
- Allergic rhinitis is represented by sneezing, nasal congestion, nasal pruritus, and rhinorrhea. When allergic disease is suspected, a skin prick test can be performed for confirmation. When skin testing is difficult to interpret or not feasible (ie, dermatographism), allergen-specific immunoglobulin (Ig) E serum testing based on the patient's history can be useful. The specific in vitro assays chosen should be based on local prevalence of aeroallergens.
- Oral antihistamines should be used to treat patients with mild or occasional seasonal allergic rhinitis. Cromolyn is an alternative to oral antihistamines in mild disease.
- The pathophysiology of nonallergic rhinitis does not involve IgE mediation. The specific mechanism is poorly understood because of the many presentations of the conditions in this category. What is known about the pathophysiology is that the nonallergic rhinitis is caused by nasal hyperactivity to nonimmunologic stimuli, but little is known regarding the exact mechanism of this nasal hyperactivity.
- Because of the variance in causes of nonallergic rhinitis, treatments also vary. Vasomotor rhinitis, nonallergic rhinitis with eosinophil syndrome, and rhinitis medicamentosa are best treated with intranasal corticosteroids. Irrigation and debridement are the standard treatment of atrophic rhinitis, with an occasional course of antibiotics if needed for acute infection. For gustatory rhinitis, pretreatment with ipratropium bromide can be used.

No financial disclosures.
No conflict of interest.
Department of Family and Community Medicine, University of Kansas School of Medicine – Wichita, 1010 North Kansas, Wichita, KS 67214, USA
E-mail address: sheryl.beard@viachristi.org

Prim Care Clin Office Pract 41 (2014) 33–46
http://dx.doi.org/10.1016/j.pop.2013.10.005
0095-4543/14/$ – see front matter © 2014 Elsevier Inc. All rights reserved.

INTRODUCTION

Rhinitis is defined as inflammation of the mucous membrane lining in the nasal passages.[1–4] Rhinitis presents as nasal congestion, sneezing, nasal and palatal itching, rhinorrhea, and postnasal drainage. The categories of rhinitis include allergic, nonallergic, and infectious. A diagnosis of rhinitis should lead the provider to consider other coexisting conditions, such as asthma.

EPIDEMIOLOGY

Rhinitis is viewed by some as a trivial disease, but it may impair work, school, daily functioning, sleeping patterns, and quality of life.[4] Fifty-eight million people have allergic rhinitis, and 19 million people have nonallergic rhinitis, in United States.[2] Twenty-six million Americans have mixed rhinitis. Mixed rhinitis has components of both allergic and nonallergic rhinitis.[2] In 2002, the estimated direct and indirect costs to society for rhinitis were nearly US$11.6 billion dollars.[4]

Seventy percent of patients with allergic disease acquire the disease in childhood, and 70% of patients with nonallergic disease acquire it in adulthood, at more than 20 years of age.[2] Nonallergic rhinitis has a female predominance.

ALLERGIC RHINITIS
Classification

No standard classification exists for rhinitis. Allergic rhinitis is classified in the literature according to its seasonality, its perennial nature, or its occupational association. Seasonal allergic rhinitis is commonly caused by a variety of pollen allergens. Perennial allergic rhinitis is mainly caused by dust mites and animal dander. Occupational rhinitis results from airborne particles in the workplace and is a response to allergic and nonallergic mechanisms. Examples of occupational allergic antigens include animals and wood dust exposure. Chemicals and other irritants are examples of occupational nonallergic antigens. Infectious rhinitis is caused by infectious agents such as rhinovirus and may be complicated by bacterial infection.

Rhinitis can also be classified by whether it is persistent, intermittent, or episodic. Persistent rhinitis lasts longer than 4 weeks or more than 4 days per week. Intermittent rhinitis is defined as symptoms that last less than 4 weeks and fewer than 4 days per week. Episodic rhinitis may occur with sporadic inhalant aeroallergen exposure not typically encountered by the patient's usual indoor and outdoor environments, such as visiting a house with pets. This article uses the seasonal, perennial, and occupational rhinitis descriptors.

Regardless of the classification terminology used, all forms of rhinitis are further characterized by their severity. Mild rhinitis is described as rhinitis that does not impair work, school, daily functioning, or sleeping patterns. Moderate to severe rhinitis interferes with quality of life and disturbs activities of daily living and/or sleep. Severe rhinitis is so marked that normal functioning cannot take place without treatment.

Pathophysiology

Allergic rhinitis is the result of an immunoglobulin (Ig) E-mediated allergic reaction, with varying degrees of nasal inflammation.[1] Allergic rhinitis results from a type I hypersensitivity response to an inhaled allergen.[5] Allergens are proteins derived from airborne particulate matter, including dust mite feces, pollens, animal dander, and cockroach particles.[5]

Antigen-presenting cells (APCs) engulf allergens in the nasal mucosa.[5] The cells break the allergens into antigenic peptides.[5] APCs present the antigenic peptides to naive T cells (Th0).[5] When activated, Th0 cells differentiate into the Th2 subtype.[5] The Th2 cells release interleukin (IL)-4, which stimulates B cells to produce IgE.[5] IgE attaches to mast cells and basophils and renders them sensitized to the allergen.[5] When sensitized, mast cells and basophil cells are exposed to the allergen, and they degranulate.[5] Degranulation of these cells releases a host of mediators including histamine and prostaglandin.[5] Mast cell release of histamine is a major pathway for nasal inflammation in seasonal and perennial allergic disease.[1] Leukotrienes, kinins, and prostaglandins also play a role in the allergic pathway.[1]

Early and late phase reactions
Allergen exposure produces symptoms within minutes of the exposure and diminishes by 1 hour. Allergic reactions consist of early phase and late phase reactions.[5] Early phase reactions involve the mediation of IgE-allergen complexes and produce the typical symptoms of allergic rhinitis.[5] Late phase reactions involve activation and sequestration of inflammatory cells that produce vascular congestion and nasal hyperresponsiveness.[5] Inflammatory cells that migrate into the nasal mucosa include eosinophils, basophils, monocytes, T cells, and neutrophils.[5] The resultant inflammation causes the normal nasal response to become exaggerated.[5] Because of the nasal hyperresponsiveness, some individuals with allergic rhinitis can experience allergic symptoms on exposure to nonallergic stimuli (such as perfumes, smoke, strong odors, or other irritants).[5]

Eosinophils play a major role in nasal hyperresponsiveness.[5] Eosinophils arrive after allergen exposure and produce IL-5. IL-5 promotes activation and survival of other eosinophils.[5] Eosinophils also release toxic products that damage local mucosal cells.[5]

Prevention

Identifying the environmental allergens or irritants that trigger rhinitis symptoms can be important in the management of the disease process.[4] Mild disease can usually be managed with avoidance measures alone.[1] Allergen removal can also improve the severity of allergic rhinitis and can reduce the need for medications.[1] Pollen, dust mites, animals, insect proteins, and fungi are the most prominent allergic triggers.[4] Environmental control may take weeks to months to produce full beneficial effects, and complete avoidance of allergen is usually not feasible or practical.[1]

Reduction of dust mite allergen exposure can be accomplished in the following ways: remove carpets and soft toys, use covers impermeable to allergens for mattresses and pillows, vacuum beds weekly, and wash bedding at 60°C (140°F).[1] Pet dander avoidance can only be effectively managed by removing the pet and carefully cleaning all carpets, furniture, and mattresses.[1]

Implementation of avoidance measures is largely based on consensus panel recommendations because of the lack of high-quality evidence.[6,7] As with any treatment regimen or avoidance strategy, subpopulations of patients may respond differently to the same treatment plan.[8] A patient's treatment plan requires individualization based on factors such as age, symptom severity, seasonality, route of medication administration preference (ie, nasal vs oral), medication side effects, cost, onset of action, and benefit to comorbid conditions.[8]

Avoidance is the first-line treatment of any form of rhinitis. The Allergic Rhinitis and its Impact on Asthma (ARIA) guidelines: 2010 Revision recommended environmental control measures for allergic rhinitis prevention (**Box 1**).[6]

Box 1
Environmental control measures for the prevention and treatment of allergic rhinitis

- Dust mite control
  - Encase bedding in dust mite covers
  - Wash bedding and toys at 60°C or hotter
  - Avoid carpets
- Eliminate or reduce occupational exposure to allergens
- Use small particulate furnace filters
- Pollen control
  - Keep windows closed
  - Use air conditioning
  - Limit outdoor exposure
- Mold control
  - Avoid basements
  - Reduce household humidity
- Pets
  - Avoid pets in the home
  - Confine pets to uncarpeted rooms
  - Bathe pets frequently
  - Equip rooms with high-efficiency particulate air filters

The ARIA guidelines make recommendations for children and pregnant or lactating women. Women should breast-feed for the first 3 months of life irrespective of atopic family history. The ARIA guidelines also state that pregnant and lactating women should not avoid food-related antigens for the prevention of childhood allergic rhinitis. In addition, children and pregnant women should completely avoid tobacco smoke exposure.[6]

Diagnosis

Allergic rhinitis is represented by sneezing, nasal congestion, nasal pruritus, and rhinorrhea.[2] When allergic disease is suspected, a skin prick test can be performed for confirmation.[1] When skin testing is difficult to interpret or not feasible (ie, dermatographism), allergen-specific IgE serum testing based on the patient's history can be useful.[1] The specific in vitro assays chosen should be based on local prevalence of aeroallergens.[4]

History

The history can be an important component in the differentiation of rhinitis. Nasal pruritus, palatal pruritus, sneezing, allergen exposure, seasonality, and associated ocular symptoms suggest allergic disease.[3,8] A family history of allergy is also an important clue that symptoms might be allergy related.[9]

Treatment

Oral antihistamines should be used to treat patients with mild or occasional seasonal allergic rhinitis. Cromolyn is an alternative to oral antihistamines in mild disease.[1]

Intranasal corticosteroids are effective in treating seasonal allergic rhinitis of moderate or long duration. If the patient's seasonal allergic rhinitis is severe, an oral antihistamine can be added to the intranasal corticosteroid. Other considerations for severe seasonal allergic rhinitis include adding oral decongestants, ipratropium bromide, or analgesics. As a last resort, immunotherapy should be considered for those who fail other therapies.[1]

Primary treatment of perennial allergic rhinitis is avoidance. Oral or intranasal antihistamines are effective for mild or intermittent symptoms not controlled with avoidance. Moderate or frequent symptoms should be treated with intranasal corticosteroids. Adding an oral antihistamine can be done if corticosteroids alone are not effective.[1]

Severe symptoms usually require additional therapies such as topical or oral decongestants for congestion and ipratropium bromide for rhinorrhea. Immunotherapy can be considered, but is not as effective in treating perennial allergic rhinitis as it is in treating seasonal allergic rhinitis.[1] As a last resort, surgical reduction of turbinate hypertrophy is an option.

Therapies not recommended by the ARIA guidelines include acupuncture, butterbur, herbal medicines, phototherapy, or other physical techniques.

NONALLERGIC RHINITIS
Classification

Nonallergic rhinitis is subdivided into several categories (**Box 2**). Nonallergic rhinitis is also known as perennial nonallergic rhinitis, idiopathic rhinitis, and vasomotor rhinitis.[3]

Box 2
Nonallergic rhinitis classification

- Vasomotor: associated with irritants and change in temperature and humidity, alcohol, exercise; involves activation of neural efferent pathway to nasal mucosa, anticholinergic mediated; may be autonomic dysfunction.

- Gustatory rhinitis: nasal congestion associated with ingestion of foods, alcoholic beverages.

- Nonallergic rhinitis with eosinophil syndrome (NARES): paroxysms of symptom flares including sneezing, watery rhinorrhea, nasal itching, congestion, and some anosmia; nasal eosinophils are present, but systemic allergy is lacking.

- Rhinitis medicamentosa: caused by prolonged and repetitive use of topical nasal decongestants. Also associated with cocaine use. Patients have rebound congestion.

- Occupational rhinitis: symptoms from irritating chemicals, grain dust, laboratory animal antigens, wood, ozone. May coexist with occupational asthma.

- Hormonal rhinitis: rhinitis related to pregnancy or the menstrual cycle. Symptoms resolve 2 weeks after delivery. Sinusitis is 6 times more common in pregnancy.

- Drug-induced rhinitis: associated with angiotensin-converting enzyme (ACE) inhibitors, phosphodiesterase-5 selective inhibitors, alpha receptor antagonists, phentolamine.

- Atrophic rhinitis: caused by glandular cell atrophy. Symptoms include nasal crusting, dryness, and fetor. Abnormally wide nasal cavities; squamous metaplasia of nasal mucosa.

- Cold air–induced rhinitis: symptoms occur on exposure to cold air.

- Anatomic rhinitis: caused by polyps, tumors, septal disturbances.

Data from Wallace D, Dykewicz M. The diagnosis and management of rhinitis: an updated practice parameter. J Allergy Clin Immunol 2008;122:S1–84.

Pathophysiology

A normal nasal response is how the nasal mucosa normally functions in response to exogenous physical stimuli. Hyperresponsiveness is the exaggeration of the normal nasal mucosa response to any stimuli. Genetic or pathologic factors can alter how the nasal mucosa functions in response to these stimuli.[5]

The pathophysiology of nonallergic rhinitis does not involve IgE mediation. The specific mechanism is poorly understood because of the many presentations of the conditions in this category.[2,3] What is known about the pathophysiology is that the nonallergic rhinitis is caused by nasal hyperactivity to nonimmunologic stimuli, but little knowledge exists regarding the exact mechanism of this nasal hyperactivity.[2] Autonomic dysregulation and nociceptive nerve dysfunction are proposed mechanisms of nasal hyperresponsiveness.[3] Because of its lack of an allergic component, nonallergic rhinitis is frequently distinguished from allergic rhinitis by negative IgE testing and/or negative skin prick testing.[2]

Diagnosis/History

The diagnosis of nonallergic rhinitis is driven by the patient's history of symptoms (see **Box 2**). Specific diagnostic tests may help clarify the diagnosis, although they are often unnecessary.

Treatment

Because of the variance in causes of nonallergic rhinitis, treatments also vary. **Box 3** summarizes specific treatments. Vasomotor rhinitis, NARES, and rhinitis medicamentosa are best treated with intranasal corticosteroids. Irrigation and debridement are the standard treatment of atrophic rhinitis, with an occasional course of antibiotics if needed for acute infection. For gustatory rhinitis, pretreatment with ipratropium bromide can be used.

LOCAL ALLERGIC RHINITIS

Local allergic rhinitis is a newly recognized subset of rhinitis. The allergic reaction of local allergic rhinitis is confined to the nose. The local inflammatory response is similar to allergic rhinitis, but a systemic response is lacking. Some patients previously classified as having nonallergic rhinitis are now being found to have local allergic rhinitis.[10] Local allergic rhinitis is confined to the nasal mucosa and is characterized by local inflammatory reactions including local infiltration of eosinophils and localized detection of IgE in response to aeroallergens.[10] Patients with local allergic rhinitis do not have

---

Box 3
Treatment of nonallergic rhinitis

1. Vasomotor rhinitis: intranasal corticosteroids
2. NARES: intranasal corticosteroids
3. Atrophic: irrigation, debridement, antibiotics as needed
4. Gustatory: ipratropium bromide
5. Occupational: avoidance
6. Hormonal: nasal saline
7. Rhinitis medicamentosa: intranasal corticosteroids or oral steroids

significant systemic reactions to aeroallergens including negative skin prick testing and negative serum IgE levels.[10] Local allergic rhinitis is associated with asthma and conjunctivitis and commonly begins in childhood.[10] The prevalence of local allergic rhinitis is unknown and its clinical relevance is unclear.[10] However, in a small study, the prevalence of local allergic rhinitis was approximately 26%.[10]

DIAGNOSTIC TESTING

Testing that can be performed in the evaluation of allergic or nonallergic rhinitis includes skin prick testing, which can be helpful to rule in or rule out allergic disease.[4] Total serum IgE or IgG levels should not be routinely performed. Total serum IgE levels have low sensitivity for predicting allergic disease. IgE testing, specific to local aeroallergens, may be indicated if skin prick testing is not feasible or is difficult to interpret, such as in a patient with dermatographism. Increased serum IgG levels have been suggested as a risk factor for atopy, but evidence has been inconclusive.[4] Nasal smears to assess for eosinophils are not recommended for routine use.[8]

Fiberoptic nasal endoscopy can be helpful, but is expensive and should be reserved for those patients with atypical symptoms or those with inadequate response to treatment.[4]

Rhinomanometry measures the airflow obstruction in the upper airway and can give the clinician an objective measurement of nasal congestion in response to certain interventions. Rhinomanometry can be useful in assessing the severity of an anatomic abnormality and assessing those patients with obstructive sleep apnea.[4] A sleep study should be considered in patients presenting with chronic rhinitis, because chronic rhinitis is a risk factor for sleep disordered breathing.[4]

Computed tomography scans and magnetic resonance imaging are expensive but can be used to identify anatomic abnormalities using coronal sections. However, this type of imaging may not correlate well with functional obstruction.[4]

Patients with watery rhinorrhea and recent nasal surgery or trauma may have a cerebrospinal fluid (CSF) leak. Beta transferrin protein testing can be performed on the rhinorrhea and can confirm a CSF leak.[4]

DIFFERENTIAL DIAGNOSIS

Diagnoses to consider when a patient presents with rhinitis are listed in **Box 4**.

Smelling difficulty may suggest nasal polyps and unilateral symptoms may signify an anatomic problem.[4,8] **Box 5** outlines questions that help in the diagnosis and classification of rhinitis and **Box 6** lists physical examination systems that should be evaluated in patients with rhinitis. Particular attention should be placed on examination of the nasal passages.

MEDICATIONS
Intranasal Corticosteroids

Intranasal corticosteroids (INCS) should be first-line treatment of allergic rhinitis in the moderate to severe category, and they are the most effective treatment of all nasal allergic rhinitis symptoms.[1,8,9] INCS are recommended in chronic rhinosinusitis.[9] There is no relevant difference between INCS preparations and no INCS preparation is more efficacious than another.[3] Budesonide is US Food and Drug Administration (FDA) indicated for the treatment of nonallergic rhinitis. The INCS mometasone has an indication for nasal polyposis.[9]

Box 4
Differential diagnosis of patients presenting with rhinitis

- Allergic rhinitis
- Nonallergic rhinitis
- Occupational rhinitis
- Structural/anatomic factors
  - Deviated septum
  - Nasal and sinus tumors
  - Nasal turbinate hypertrophy
  - Nasal polyposis
- CSF rhinorrhea
- Pharyngonasal reflux
- Infectious rhinitis
  - Rhinovirus
  - Coronavirus
  - Bacterial infection
- Chronic sinusitis
- Ciliary dyskinesia syndrome
- Systemic disorders
  - Wegener disease
  - Tuberculosis
  - Syphilis
- Medication side effects
  - ACE inhibitors
  - Phosphodiesterase-5 selective inhibitors
  - Alpha receptor antagonists
  - Phentolamine
- Hormonal disturbances
- Aspirin intolerance
- Exogenous noxious stimuli
- Rhinitis sicca (chronically dry mucous membranes)
- Atrophic rhinitis
- Local allergic rhinitis
- Rhinitis medicamentosa
- Vasomotor rhinitis
- Gustatory rhinitis
- NARES
- Cold air–induced rhinitis

Data from van Cauwenberge P, Bachert C, Passalacqua G, et al. Consensus statement on the treatment of allergic rhinitis. European Academy of Allergology and Clinical Immunology. Allergy 2000;55:116–34; and Wallace D, Dykewicz M. The diagnosis and management of rhinitis: an updated practice parameter. J Allergy Clin Immunol 2008;122:S1–84.

Box 5
Components of the history important to consider when evaluating the patient with rhinitis

- Pattern (perennial, seasonal, or combination)
- Triggers
- Family history
- Current medications
- Previous response to treatment
- Comorbid conditions
- Environmental history
- Occupational exposures

Data from Wallace D, Dykewicz M. The diagnosis and management of rhinitis: an updated practice parameter. J Allergy Clin Immunol 2008;122:S1–84.

Side effects of INCS include nasal burning, irritation, stinging, epistaxis, and local dryness.[3] Mucosal atrophy is not a noted side effect. Local candidiasis is rarely seen with INCS use.[3] INCS have negligible hypothalamic-pituitary-adrenal axis suppression and the systemic burden of intranasal corticosteroids is clinically insignificant.[3]

The mechanism of action of INCS involves the reduction of the inflammatory response. Glucocorticoids move through the outer cellular membrane, binding to intracellular receptors.[3] Intracellular steroid complexes are transported to the cell nucleus where responsive genes are either upregulated or downregulated.[3] Gene modulation leads to a reduction in proinflammatory mediators in the mucosa.[3]

Oral Antihistamines

Oral antihistamines reduce nasal itching, rhinorrhea, and sneezing but do not treat nasal congestion effectively.[1] Oral antihistamines can reduce conjunctivitis and urticaria.[1]

First-generation oral antihistamines are poorly selective for H-1 receptors and can cause anticholinergic effects by blocking muscarinic receptors. Blockade of the muscarinic receptors causes dry mucous membranes, blurry vision, constipation, tachycardia, and urinary retention.[3] Because first-generation antihistamines cross the blood-brain barrier, significant sedation occurs.[3] The sedative effects of these antihistamines have been linked to industrial accidents and contribute to significant loss of function at work and school.[3] Overall, first-generation antihistamines are limited in usefulness because of these sedative and anticholinergic effects.[3]

Second-generation antihistamines have better selectivity for the H-1 receptor.[3] A more complex molecular structure allows second-generation antihistamines to not cross the blood-brain barrier. These antihistamines are considered nonsedating.[9] The risk/benefit ratio of second-generation antihistamines is so favorable that they are considered first-line therapy for mild allergic rhinitis. Tolerance to antihistamines has not been shown to occur.

Intranasal Antihistamines

Azelastine 0.1% has an indication for allergic and vasomotor rhinitis and is the only nasal antihistamine available in the United States.[3] Intranasal antihistamine (INA)

Box 6
Systemic physical examination of patient with rhinitis

- General
  - Elongated facies
  - Mouth breathing
- Ears
  - Tympanic membrane
    - Air fluid level
    - Erythema
    - Retraction
    - Mobility
- Nose
  - External crease
- Nasal mucosa[2]
  - Bluish discoloration
  - Red nasal mucosa
  - Excessive watery-clear mucus
  - Polyps
  - Chronic sinusitis
  - Turbinate hypertrophy
  - Crusting
  - Discharge
  - Septal deviation
  - Septal perforation
- Eyelids
  - Venous stasis of the lower lids (allergic shiners)
- Conjunctiva
  - Edema
  - Erythema
  - Excessive lacrimation
  - Cobblestoning
- Oropharynx
  - High-arch palate
  - Tonsillar enlargement
  - Adenoid enlargement
  - Cobblestoning
- Neck
  - Thyroid examination
  - Lymphadenopathy

- Respiratory
  - Wheezing
- Abdomen
  - Liver enlargement
  - Spleen enlargement
- Skin
  - Eczema
  - Urticaria
  - Dermatographism

Data from Wallace D, Dykewicz M. The diagnosis and management of rhinitis: an updated practice parameter. J Allergy Clin Immunol 2008;122:S1–84.

may be better than oral antihistamines in reducing total nasal symptom scores.[3] Nasal antihistamines can help control nasal congestion.[9]

Side effects of intranasal antihistamines include bitter taste, headache, epistaxis, and nasal irritation.[3,9] Nasal antihistamines do not produce a significant amount of sedation.[1] INA has the advantage of a quicker onset of action for nasal and ocular symptoms compared with INCS.[1]

Nasal antihistamines need to be administered twice daily for maximum clinical benefit.[1]

Intranasal Ipratropium

Intranasal ipratropium (IP) controls seromucous gland secretion by blocking muscarinic receptors, so it is effective in treating watery rhinorrhea.[1] IP is useful in treating nonallergic rhinitis and the common cold.[1] Ipratropium does not improve nasal congestion or sneezing.[1] Side effects of IP include nasal dryness, burning, irritation, stuffy nose, headache, and dry mouth.[1]

Because of its onset of action, nasal anticholinergics (ipratropium) as well as nasal corticosteroids, nasal antihistamines, and oral antihistamines, are effective in the treatment of episodic allergic rhinitis.[8]

Leukotriene Receptor Antagonists

Montelukast is the only leukotriene receptor antagonist (LTRA) that is FDA approved for allergic rhinitis treatment, but it has a limited role in nonallergic rhinitis.[3] LTRAs should be used as second-line or third-line therapy[3] and should not be used in those patients with episodic symptoms.[8]

Nasal Cromolyn

Nasal cromolyn can be used before allergen exposure for prophylaxis of episodic allergic rhinitis.[9] Cromolyn should be considered for early mild rhinitis, but should not be considered a first-line treatment in allergic rhinitis.[1] Nasal cromolyn is mostly void of side effects. It should be administered 3 to 4 times a day.[1,9] The mechanism of action is poorly understood, but evidence suggests that it inhibits mast cell degranulation.[9]

Decongestants

Oral and topical decongestants may be used for symptomatic relief in patients with nonallergic rhinitis.[3] Oral and topical decongestants affect the alpha adrenoreceptors on nasal capacitance blood vessels.[3] Nasal capacitance blood vessels are responsible for mucosal swelling resulting in nasal congestion.[3] Oral decongestants act on the sympathetic tone of blood vessels through the adrenergic pathway causing vasoconstriction.[1]

Topical phenylephrine and topical oxymetazoline are over-the-counter topical decongestants.[9] Topical decongestants are effective in treatment of nasal congestion, but should not be used for more than 5 days because of the risk of rebound vasodilatation, and subsequent rebound congestion (rhinitis medicamentosa).[1,9] Tolerance may be prevented by concurrent use of INCS.[3]

Side effects of topical decongestants are stinging, burning, dryness, and mucosal ulceration (less common).[3] Oral decongestant side effects include insomnia, anxiety and tremors, tachycardia, increases in blood pressure, and palpitations.[3] Oral decongestants should be not be used in young children and adults more than 60 years of age.[1]

Combination Therapies

Combination therapy may provide a therapeutic advantage, but cost must be considered and it may reduce compliance.[8] Fluticasone with azelastine is superior to INCS alone for moderate-severe allergic rhinitis.[3,8,9] Oral antihistamines with oral decongestants are more effective than antihistamines alone for nasal congestion relief.[8]

Intranasal anticholinergics and intranasal corticosteroid combination therapy is more effective for relief of rhinorrhea than either drug as monotherapy.[8] Although inferior to intranasal corticosteroid treatment, an oral antihistamine with montelukast has an additive effect for the treatment of allergic rhinitis.[3]

Nasal Saline

Nasal saline plays a role in allergic and nonallergic rhinitis by promoting ciliary clearance, and removing mucus and other irritant materials.[3] Some evidence suggests that hypertonic saline provides modest benefit compared with isotonic saline.[3]

Anti-IgE

Omalizumab is a monoclonal antibody available for the treatment of poorly controlled asthma, but it might have a role in the treatment of allergic rhinitis.[3] Omalizumab has proven efficacy in allergic rhinitis, but is limited because of high cost, anaphylaxis reports, and availability in only injectable form.[3]

Omalizumab binds to IgE and hinders its relationship with inflammatory cells.[3] Omalizumab only binds to circulating IgE and not bound IgE.[3]

Systemic Steroids

Systemic steroids should not be used as first-line treatment of allergic rhinitis. The risk of adverse effects of systemic steroids precludes using them for longer than 3 weeks. Systemic steroids should not be used in children or pregnant women. Because few studies are available to support the use of systemic steroids, they are used as a last resort.[1]

Immunotherapy

Subcutaneous immunotherapy

Subcutaneous immunotherapy (SCIT) involves the subcutaneous injection of aqueous extracts of an offending allergen. By starting at low doses of the injected allergen and by progressively increasing the dose, SCIT builds up immunity to the offending allergen.[11] SCIT is indicated for adults and children presenting with pollen-induced and dust mite–induced allergic rhinitis, and in those patients for whom medications and avoidance measures are inadequate.[11] SCIT is the only treatment that has proved to alter the course of allergic disease.[9] Evidence suggests that immunotherapy can halt the advancement of allergic disease that causes asthma and that it halts the creation of new sensitivities.[11] Children, patients early in the disease process, and patients with few sensitivities are the most likely to benefit from SCIT.[11]

SCIT starts with a buildup phase, which entails increasing the injected allergen dose over time. When the maximum dose of allergen extract is reached, the maintenance phase begins.[1] The maximum dose of allergen in the injections is variable among the different allergen extracts. For example, the maximum dose of dust mite allergen is 7 μg.[11] The usual recommendation is that maintenance treatment should last for 3 years.[11] After an average of 3 to 4 years of maintenance immunotherapy, the effectiveness of treatment lasts for 3 years or more after discontinuation.[11]

The inherent risk of SCIT is systemic anaphylaxis.[1,11] The rate of significant systemic reactions in patients with allergic rhinitis is approximately 5%.[1] Times of the year with increased pollen count can predispose to severe and life-threatening systemic reactions to SCIT.[11] Patients must wait 20 to 30 minutes after SCIT treatment to monitor for severe reactions.[11] Pretreatment with antihistamines has the potential to reduce systemic reactions.[11]

MONITORING

The Total Nasal Symptoms Score is a subjective assessment of a patients' specific symptoms, including rhinorrhea, nasal congestion, sneezing, and pruritus, and can be used to assess effectiveness of medications.[8] The Rhinoconjunctivitis Quality of Life Questionnaire is another tool that can be used for monitoring of therapy.[8] Based on the results of the screening tool used, the provider should consider stepping down treatment when the patients' symptoms have been controlled.[8]

Consultation with an allergist is based on several factors. Patients under evaluation for allergy testing and immunotherapy should be considered for consultation with an allergist/immunologist. Other instances in which a consultation might be considered is if a patient has a severe and prolonged course of rhinitis; if there are comorbid conditions present, such as asthma, chronic sinusitis, or nasal polyps; or if symptoms are interfering with quality of life or ability to function.[4]

INFECTIOUS RHINITIS/RHINOSINUSITIS

Infectious rhinitis and rhinosinusitis are synonymous with sinusitis. Acute rhinosinusitis most commonly occurs as a complication of viral upper respiratory infections.[9] Viral upper respiratory infections cause mucosal edema leading to obstruction of the sinus openings as well as ciliary function impairment.[9] The low-oxygen environment and the stagnant mucus of the sinuses allow viral and bacterial proliferation.[9]

Chronic rhinosinusitis is the result of long-term obstruction and/or function of the sinuses.[9] Chronic inflammation of the nasal mucosa leads to chronic low-grade infections.[9]

REFERENCES

1. van Cauwenberge P, Bachert C, Passalacqua G, et al. Consensus statement on the treatment of allergic rhinitis. European Academy Allergology Clinical Immunology. Allergy 2000;55:116–34.

2. Settipane R, Charnock D. Epidemiology of rhinitis: allergic and nonallergic. Clin Allergy Immunol 2007;19:23–34.
3. Greiner A, Meltzer E. Overview of the treatment of allergic rhinitis and nonallergic rhinopathy. Proc Am Thorac Soc 2011;8:121–31.
4. Wallace D, Dykewicz M. The diagnosis and management of rhinitis: an updated practice parameter. J Allergy Clin Immunol 2008;122:S1–84.
5. Sin B, Togias A. Pathophysiology of allergic and nonallergic rhinitis. Proc Am Thorac Soc 2011;8:106–14.
6. Brozek J, Bousquet J, Baena-Cagnani C, et al. Allergic rhinitis and its impact on asthma (ARIA) guidelines: 2010 revision. J Allergy Clin Immunol 2010;126(3): 466–76.
7. Cox L, Compalati E, Canonica W. Will sublingual immunotherapy become an approved treatment method in the United States? Curr Allergy Asthma Rep 2011;11(1):4–6.
8. Dykewicz M. Management of rhinitis: guidelines, evidence basis, and systematic clinical approach for what we do. Immunol Allergy Clin North Am 2011;31: 619–34.
9. Chaaban M, Corey J. Pharmacotherapy of rhinitis and rhinosinusitis. Facial Plast Surg Clin North Am 2012;20:61–71.
10. Rondon C, Campo P, Galindo L, et al. Prevalence and clinic relevance of local allergic rhinitis. Allergy 2012. http://dx.doi.org/10.1111/all.12002.
11. Wu AY. Immunotherapy–vaccines for allergic disease. J Thorac Dis 2012;4(2): 198–202.

Rhinosinusitis

Alexi DeCastro, MD[a,b], Lisa Mims, MD[a], William J. Hueston, MD[c],*

KEYWORDS

- Rhinosinusitis • Terminology • Diagnostic criteria • Imaging • Treatment

KEY POINTS

- Sinusitis affects 1 in 7 adults each year and, even although it is common, controversy still exists regarding terminology, diagnostic criteria, indications for imaging, and treatment guidelines.
- Disease develops secondary to increased mucus production, decreased ciliary function, and subsequent obstruction of the ostiomeatal complex. Patients then present with symptoms of nasal congestion, purulent nasal discharge, and sinus tenderness suggestive of sinusitis.
- Although most are caused by viral infections, acute bacterial sinusitis can be diagnosed when symptoms persist for longer than 10 days, or 3 to 5 days for severe symptoms, or worsen after a period of improvement. Typical offending organisms include *Streptococcus pneumoniae* and *Haemophilus influenzae*, but may include other respiratory pathogens, which should be considered based on the patient history and risk factors.
- Routine radiographic imaging is not recommended for diagnostic purposes and should be used only in cases of suspected complications.
- Patients who are diagnosed with bacterial sinusitis should be started on amoxicillin-clavulanate unless an allergy is reported, in which case doxycycline or a respiratory fluoroquinolone is indicated, and treatment should be continued for 5 to 7 days in adults and 10 to 14 days in children.
- Patients who fail to respond to antibiotic therapy should be suspected of having chronic sinusitis. These patients are more likely to have irreversible changes in their nasal and paranasal structures, which require additional therapy, including endoscopic surgery.
- Referral of these patients to an otolaryngologist for further evaluation is recommended. In addition, patients with suspected fungal sinusitis should be referred to an otolaryngologist acutely, because this condition has high mortality if not treated emergently.

INTRODUCTION

Sinusitis is one of the most common conditions diagnosed and managed by primary care physicians. The cost of providing care to patients with sinusitis is estimated to be

---

[a] Department of Family Medicine, Medical University of South Carolina, 5 Charleston Center, Suite 263, MSC 192, Charleston, SC 29415-0192, USA; [b] Department of Family Medicine, MUSC Family Medicine Center, 560 Ellis Oaks Drive, Charleston, SC 29425-0192, USA; [c] Department of Family Medicine, Medical College of Wisconsin, 8701 Watertown Plank Road, PO Box 26509, Milwaukee, WI 53226, USA
* Corresponding author.
E-mail address: whueston@mcw.edu

Prim Care Clin Office Pract 41 (2014) 47–61
http://dx.doi.org/10.1016/j.pop.2013.10.006 **primarycare.theclinics.com**

$3 billion per year just in the United States,[1] and it is the fifth most common condition for which antibiotics are prescribed. Clearly, this is a medical problem that most primary care physicians encounter on a daily basis, so an understanding of the pathophysiology of this illness, how to most efficiently diagnose the problems, and judicious use of antibiotics are essential when caring for these patients.

Furthermore, despite the frequency at which sinusitis is diagnosed and treated, several controversies persist regarding the accurate diagnosis of this condition and the most appropriate management strategies. Debates about the usefulness of imaging studies and when these might be helpful, the predictive accuracy of the constellation of clinical signs and symptoms that might differentiate sinusitis from other upper respiratory conditions, such as allergic rhinitis and common cold, and the effectiveness of antibiotics in treating acute sinusitis continue to cloud the clinical approach to this common problem.

Adding to the uncertainty for clinicians is the inclusion of acute sinusitis into the less specific condition called rhinosinusitis, which includes other upper respiratory conditions, such as common cold. The inclusion of acute sinusitis with common cold and other upper respiratory conditions is partly justified by the difficulty in discerning one from the other. Because there is sinus inflammation even in viral upper respiratory tract conditions, there is some justification in combining these 2 infectious processes into a single entity. However, the use of this less specific diagnostic category may offer justification for clinicians to prescribe antibiotics for patients with common colds by citing evidence that this treatment works for sinusitis. In this review, studies are isolated that focus only on patients with either the clinical characteristics that have been linked independently to sinus inflammation, apart from concomitant nasal inflammation or obstruction, or that rely on other diagnostic testing to validate that the sinuses are the primary cause of the patient's complaints.

Acute Versus Chronic Sinusitis

In addition to the confusion surrounding the accuracy of diagnosing acute sinusitis is the ambiguity regarding at what point acute sinusitis should be reclassified as chronic sinusitis. The simplest criterion for this designation is the number of days that the patient has been ill, such as that propagated by the American Academy of Otolaryngology-Head and Neck Surgery, which defines chronic sinusitis as a sinus problem that persists more than 8 weeks.[1] However, this criterion is also the most arbitrary, because an overlap would be expected in patients whose symptoms are acute and would resolve with little additional diagnostic or treatment intensity as opposed to those whose problems are unlikely to resolve without further intervention.

As suggested earlier, instead of the time of illness, a more functional definition is one that conveys a different type of pathologic condition or process that indicates a shift in the diagnostic and treatment approach, as supported by Weinberg and colleagues[2] in their study of children with recurrent acute sinusitis as opposed to those with chronic sinusitis. In this study, children classified by clinical presentation and imaging as having acute sinusitis were more likely to respond to antibiotic therapy (96% vs 40% of those classified as chronic sinusitis), whereas those with chronic sinusitis more often needed surgical interventions (40% vs 6% of those diagnosed with recurrent acute sinusitis). For the purposes of this review, acute and chronic sinusitis are used to indicate when the symptoms are related to reversible changes in the nasal passages and paranasal structures (acute sinusitis), as opposed to remodeling of these structures because of long-standing inflammation or allergies, in which additional interventions are likely needed to clear the obstruction (chronic sinusitis).

PATHOPHYSIOLOGY OF SINUSITIS
Normal Sinus Anatomy and Function

The sinuses constitute a collection of facial bony cavities that interconnect with the nose through several ostia. The sinuses are lined with ciliated pseudostratified columnar epithelium and blanketed with a layer of protective mucus, which traps materials that are inhaled into the sinuses. The pulsations of the cilia across the epithelial lining propel the mucus toward the respective sinus ostium and into the nose for disposal.

The ostia for the frontal, maxillary, and anterior ethmoid sinuses all share a common connection with the nose, called the ostiomeatal complex. This complex lies in the medial nasal meatus lateral to the middle turbinate. In contrast, the posterior ethmoid and sphenoid sinuses open into the superior meatus (posterior and ethmoid) and sphenoethmoid recess (sphenoid) spaces. In contrast to the aforementioned sinuses that share the ostiomeatal complex, the ostia for the posterior ethmoid and sphenoid sinuses are more posterior in the nose and not contiguous with the middle turbinate. This anatomy offers greater protection to these sinuses from occlusion, resulting in fewer instances of sinus problems in these 2 cavities.

Sinus Disease

In most cases of sinusitis, a disturbance in the shape or function of the middle turbinate can obstruct the opening to the ostiomeatal complex, resulting in occlusion and trapping of the protective mucous blanket that coats the facial sinuses that share this passageway. These disruptions can be from mechanical insults (such as a deviated septum or trauma), medication effects (such as withdrawal from α-agonists or rhinitis medicamentosa), other noninfectious mediators (such as allergies or pregnancy), or infections (such as viruses). In addition, patients with congenital conditions that results in ciliary dysfunction, such as cystic fibrosis, Young syndrome or Kartagener syndrome, are at higher risk for sinus disease, as a result of the accumulation of thickened mucus that is contaminated with inhaled microbes and other materials.

Sinus disease develops when there is a direct insult to the sinus epithelium, resulting in excessive production of mucus, which impairs ciliary transport, along with inflammatory edema to the ostia, resulting in a trapping of the mucus within the sinus cavity. The resulting decrease in oxygen penetration in to the sinus causes relative sinus hypoxia and acidosis, resulting in further sinus epithelial irritation and destruction.[3]

With chronic inflammation, the histology of the sinus epithelium changes. Nearly a third of the usual ciliated epithelial cells may undergo metaplastic changes and become mucus-secreting cells, leading to additional sinus congestion and decreased clearing of secretions. Furthermore, the ciliary beating frequency is reduced by more than 50% from its usual frequency of 700 beats per minutes to approximately 300 beats per minute.[4] The reduction in beat frequency further reduces the effectiveness of sinus mucus clearance. With ongoing inflammation, the sinus epithelial layer becomes more edematous and balloons into the cavity, trapping the material and causing further hypoxia and acidosis.[5] These changes lead to irreversible sinus damage, such as polyps, which do not respond to acute treatments such as antibiotics.

Clinical Signs and Symptoms of Sinusitis

Because acute sinusitis complicates many other upper respiratory conditions, such as common colds or allergic rhinitis, it is difficult to differentiate the signs and symptoms that indicate sinus involvement from the complaints of patients who have rhinitis alone. In 1 study,[6] a chart review of 734 patients seen by family physicians in the United

States, 4 clinical cues (sinus tenderness, sinus pressure, postnasal drainage, and purulent drainage) were most often associated with the diagnosis of sinusitis as opposed to a cold. A similar British study[7] showed that clinicians relied on a history of sinusitis along with 3 findings to make a diagnosis of sinusitis; these were rhinorrhea, sinus tenderness, and the presence of purulent secretions. In both these studies, only one of the identified clinical conditions was independently associated with sinus infections.

Various sources define acute sinusitis as a purulent discharge of more than 10 days duration but lasting fewer than 4 weeks.[1] This definition has been proposed by the American Academy of Otolaryngology-Head and Neck Surgery and is consistent with that of the American College of Physicians (ACP). Both the American Academy of Family Physicians and the Infectious Diseases Society of America (IDSA) have endorsed the ACP definition. However, the 7-day minimum duration of symptoms has considerable overlap with uncomplicated colds, which can last 10 to 12 days.[8] In addition, patients may show other signs and symptoms consistent with bacterial infection, yet according to clinical guidelines, would not be diagnosed until they reach the temporal cutoff for acute sinusitis. Consequently, clinicians often make this diagnosis earlier than recommended.

Sinusitis or Common Cold?

Several studies have attempted to identify the key clinical signs and symptoms that are associated with sinusitis as opposed to a common cold. One drawback to all of these studies is that the gold standard for bacterial infection of the sinuses (ie, sinus aspiration and culture) is rarely performed. In the absence of this standard, most investigators have relied on positive imaging studies as a proxy for culture-proven infection. As pointed out by Williams and Simel,[9] a 4-view sinus film that has 6 mm of sinus thickening or sinus opacification has 72% to 90% accuracy for bacterial sinusitis.

With that caveat in mind, investigators have identified 5 clinical cues, 1 illness timing event, and 2 laboratory findings as independent predictors of sinusitis as opposed to a common cold. In a study by Williams and Simel,[9] 5 clinical signs and symptoms were associated with sinusitis (**Table 1**). These signs and symptoms included a history of maxillary toothache (positive likelihood ratio [PLR] = 2.5, meaning that patients with this sign were 2.5 times more likely to have sinusitis than those without it), purulent secretions (PLR = 2.1), a poor response to decongestants (PLR = 2.1), abnormal transillumination (PLR = 1.6), and a history of purulent nasal drainage (PLR = 1.5). If 4 or 5 of these factors were present, the patient was 6.4 times more likely to have sinusitis than a cold. However, if only 2 or fewer were present, then, the patient was no

Table 1			
Independent criteria for diagnosis of acute sinusitis			
Clinical Factor	Sensitivity (%)	Specificity (%)	Positive Likelihood Ratio
Maxillary toothache	11	93	2.5
Observed purulent discharge	62	67	2.1
Poor response to decongestant	—	—	2.1
Absence of transillumination	—	—	1.6
History of purulent discharge	72	52	1.5
Double sickening	72	65	2.1
Increased ESR and CRP level	82	57	—

Abbreviations: CRP, C-reactive protein; ESR, erythrocyte sedimentation rate.

more likely to have sinusitis than a cold. The absence of all of these factors meant that the patient was 10 times more likely to have a cold than sinusitis.

Using a similar standard to diagnose sinusitis, Lindbaeck and colleagues[10] identified an additional historical factor that was associated with acute sinusitis. These investigators found that patients who stated that they became ill with a respiratory ailment, then became sicker (termed double sickening), were twice as likely to have sinusitis. The presumed onset of the double sickening is believed to correspond to the bacterial infection in the obstructed sinuses, which commenced several days after the initial nasal viral infection. In a study looking at laboratory markers for sinusitis, Hansen and colleagues[11] found that increases in the erythrocyte sedimentation rate and C-reactive protein level corresponded with a positive culture of a nasal aspirate in patients with suspected acute sinusitis.

Chronic Versus Acute Sinusitis

As noted earlier, some groups differentiate chronic versus acute sinusitis solely by time. One consensus panel advocates 8 weeks as the cutoff between acute and chronic sinusitis, whereas other authorities have suggested 3 months. Because the transition from acute infection to the chronic changes that lead to irreversible epithelial damage and restructuring of the sinus is an evolving situation, it is likely arbitrary to designate 1 particular time as the juncture at which acute becomes chronic. Rather, it is more reasonable to define chronic and acute in terms of the change in symptoms and response to therapy that occur once sinus remodeling has reached a point at which the usual therapies for acute sinusitis are no longer effective.

Chronic sinusitis may be associated with a greater number and severity of systemic symptoms than acute sinusitis. Patients may complain of evening/night fevers, fatigue, and nonspecific body aches rather than symptoms that refer to the head or nose. In addition, patients with nonbacterial illnesses, such as chronic allergies, may be more likely to experience unrelenting sinus symptoms if their underlying illness if not adequately controlled.

Microbiology in Sinusitis

When bacterial infection is involved with sinusitis, the offending bacteria are those most commonly seen in other respiratory tract infections such as otitis media. In patients with acute sinusitis, *Streptococcus pneumoniae* and *Haemophilus influenzae* are the 2 most common organisms, with *Branhamella catarrhalis* seen more commonly in children.[3] Because of the hypoxic and acidotic environment in chronic sinusitis, anaerobes are much more common, with *H influenza* and *S pneumoniae* less common. In patients with chronic obstruction from nasal polyps or chronic mucociliary dysfunction such as cystic fibrosis, *Pseudomonas aeruginosa* should also be considered. Treatment duration may need to be lengthened to allow for penetration of medications to the obstructed sinus.

An additional functional criterion to differentiate the 2 conditions is that despite appropriate antibiotic therapy for prolonged treatment periods, patients with chronic sinusitis may not respond. In these cases, the obstructed ostium may need to be surgically opened to provide relief.

EPIDEMIOLOGY OF SINUSITIS
Frequency

Depending on the definition, sinusitis is either extremely common or surprisingly rare. For example, if one simply looks for thickening of the sinus epithelial layer in imaging studies, then is it estimated that approximately 40% of people who are referred for intracranial imaging for neurologic symptoms have been classified as meeting the radiologic definition of sinusitis.[12] However, most of these individuals have no symptoms at all suggestive of a sinus condition. On the other hand, only a few (0.5%–1.0%) patients who contract the common cold develop symptoms consistent with sinusitis. So even in this common condition, clinical sinusitis is rare.

Approximately 1 in 7 people suffer with acute sinusitis on an annual basis.[1] Adults are more likely to have the maxillary and anterior ethmoid sinuses involved in acute sinusitis, whereas in children, the posterior ethmoidal and sphenoid sinuses are more often affected.[13] Sinusitis is also likely to be a comorbid condition with otitis media in children.[12]

Risk Factors for Sinusitis

Risk factors include allergic rhinitis and viral upper respiratory tract infections. Consequently, acute sinusitis is more common during seasons when allergies are more prevalent and colds are common, such as autumn and winter. Patients with abnormal facial anatomy (such as a deviated septum), corrective nasal surgery (such as cleft palate repairs), and congenital conditions that impair the clearance of sinus mucus (such as cystic fibrosis or Young syndrome) are at higher risk for acute and chronic sinusitis. Patients with severe or poorly treated allergic rhinitis are also at higher risk of developing nasal polyps, which can lead to chronic sinusitis.

DIAGNOSIS

The diagnosis of acute sinusitis is based on clinical signs and symptoms. There are evidence-based guidelines to help the clinician properly diagnose and treat and avoid improper use of antimicrobial therapy. However, as stated earlier, there is some controversy about the diagnostic accuracy of these guidelines. Still, this collection of clinical signs and symptoms may help distinguish sinusitis from other upper respiratory conditions, such as allergic symptoms, or other upper respiratory infections, such as the common cold.

The terms sinusitis and rhinosinusitis are used by some clinicians interchangeably. However, the latter term is favored because the nasal mucosa is concurrently affected, and it is uncommon for sinusitis to occur without rhinitis.[14] Symptoms may consist of nasal congestion and obstruction, purulent nasal discharge, maxillary tooth pain, facial pain, fever, ear pressure or fullness, and headache.

Classification on Sinusitis

Sinusitis is classified temporally. Acute rhinosinusitis (ARS) is described as symptoms for less than 4 weeks, subacute rhinosinusitis, from 4 to 8 weeks, and then chronic rhinosinusitis, which persists for greater than 8 weeks. Recurrent ARS is diagnosed after 4 or more episodes of ARS per year, with interim symptom resolution.[15] Rhinosinusitis may also be classified according to site (ie, maxillary, ethmoid, sphenoid, frontal).

Physical Examination Findings

Physical examination should include assessment for upper respiratory infections: examining the eyes, ears, pharynx, teeth, sinus tenderness, lymph nodes, and chest. Direct percussion of the sinuses may not be helpful in diagnosis. A more reliable physical examination maneuver is when pain is localized to the sinuses when the patient is told to bend forward.[16] A handheld otoscope with a nasal speculum may be used for anteriɑɪ ɪlɪnɒscopy, which may identify purulent nasal discharge, rhinorrhea, mucosal edema, or nasal turbinate swelling. Nasal polyps and septal deviation are other anatomic findings that may increase the patient's risk for developing ARS.

Differentiating Bacterial from Viral Sinusitis

Clinical presentation has disappointingly limited accuracy to differentiate viral rhinosinusitis from secondary bacterial infection.[17] Numerous clinical criteria have been recommended to help distinguish bacterial and viral infection. In a review of studies for the predictive value of these clinical criteria in diagnosing acute bacterial rhinosinusitis (ABRS),[18] none proved their validity with bacterial culture in sinus aspirates. The diagnosis of ARS is nevertheless based on clinical signs and symptoms. No further diagnostic testing is needed when evaluating sinusitis without signs or symptoms of a more complicated disease process. The 2 criteria found to be most highly predictive of ARS are purulent rhinorrhea, nasal congestion and facial pain pressure fullness, or both.[1] Other symptoms, such as cough, headache, ear fullness, or loss of smell, may add more validity to the clinical diagnosis.

Thus, the diagnosis of viral rhinosinusitis is based on the symptoms, length of disease, and progression, which is the natural history of the rhinovirus. Partial or complete resolution of symptoms within 7 to 10 days after the onset of an upper respiratory tract infection suggests a cause of acute viral rhinosinusitis.[1,19] The classic triad for ABRS in adults (headache, facial pain, fever) is uncommon.[18] Criteria to distinguish bacterial and viral rhinosinusitis were established by a 2001 panel organized by the US Centers for Disease Control, which included input from several medical organizations.[20] In 2012, newer evidence-based criteria were developed by the IDSA. They recognized that only 60% of adults with symptoms persisting for 7 to 10 days have a bacterial cause identified when sinus aspirate is performed.[18] These criteria are listed in **Box 1**.

Use of Imaging in Acute Sinusitis

Imaging is not necessary in the initial diagnostic workup of ARS. Plain films are commonly ordered because of low cost, familiarity, and ease of access. However, the sensitivity and specificity of plain sinus radiography are poor for detecting mucosal thickening of the paranasal sinuses.[21] Acute radiographs are indicated only in complicated ABRS. Signs and symptoms suggesting complicated disease may include severe pain or headache, visual changes, periorbital edema, and mental status changes. If indicated, the modality of choice is the computed tomography (CT) scan, and noncontrast CT scans are indicated for recurrent or chronic sinusitis. Contrast CT may be used when there is suspicion for periorbital cellulitis or intracranial

---

Box 1
IDSA 2012 diagnostic criteria for ABRS

- Persistent symptoms or signs of ARS lasting 10 days or more without evidence of clinical improvement. Persistent symptoms commonly involve nasal discharge, whereas the presence of fever, headache, or facial pain is more variable.

- Onset of severe symptoms or signs of high fever (>39°C [102°F]) and purulent nasal discharge or facial pain for at least 3 to 4 consecutive days at the beginning of illness.

- Onset with worsening symptoms or signs (new-onset fever, headache, nasal discharge) after a typical viral upper respiratory infection that lasted 5 to 6 days and were initially improving (double sickening).

infection. Magnetic resonance imaging (MRI) is used in conjunction with CT only when there is extra sinus involvement to evaluate orbital or intracranial complications of ABRS (**Table 2**).

TREATMENT
General Management Recommendations

Management of ARS should include symptomatic and supportive care for the treatment of nasal obstruction and rhinorrhea. Pain relief with nonsteroidal antiinflammatory drugs (NSAIDs) or acetaminophen is typically used. Saline irrigation may also be used to in conjunction with NSAIDs to improve overall patient comfort. Intranasal corticosteroids may help decrease mucosal edema, thereby allowing improved sinus drainage. However, in a study by Williamson and colleagues,[22] patients with milder symptoms were the only group who benefited from topical steroids. It was theorized that the thicker nasal secretions could affect the absorption of nasal steroids because of the severity of the illness. Therefore, nasal steroids may aid in the relief of symptoms in ARS but are most helpful for patients with underlying allergic rhinitis.

The use of topical and oral decongestants, which are over the counter, may also assist in supportive care. Recent guidelines advise that they are not helpful in patients with ABRS.[18] However, if topical decongestants are used, they should be used for no more than 3 consecutive days in order to avoid rebound congestion and long-term complications like rhinitis medicamentosa. Antihistamines are used to promote symptom relief secondary to their anticholinergic drying properties, but studies have shown limited efficacy for this.[1] In addition, the drying effects of antihistamines may slow mucus transport and worsen the condition. Therefore, the routine use of antihistamines for acute sinusitis is not recommended.[18]

Management of Presumed Bacterial Sinusitis

According to the IDSA recommendations, when the diagnosis of bacterial sinusitis is confirmed per clinical guidelines (≥10 days of symptoms: purulent rhinorrhea, nasal congestion, and facial pressure), the patient should be treated with antimicrobial therapy. However, it is also recommended that certain patients with mild symptoms (only mild pain and temperature <38.3°C [101°F]) may be managed conservatively and

Table 2
Diagnostic recommendations for ARS

Modality	Indications
CT scan without contrast	Severe symptoms: visual acuity, diplopia, periorbital edema, severe headache, or altered mental status Recurrent or treatment-resistant sinusitis Rule out sinusitis (consider allergic or nonallergic rhinitis, atypical facial pain in the absence of radiologic evidence of air-fluid levels or mucosal edema)
MRI	May be used in conjunction with CT for the evaluation if extrasinus involvement is suspected (orbital or intracranial complications of ABRS)
Sinus cultures	Cultures (obtained by endoscopy) in patients with sinusitis who are not responding to empirical antibiotic therapy or suspicion of intracranial infection (acute fulminant invasive fungal rhinosinusitis, see section on complications, discussed in this article)

should be observed for a period of 7 days after diagnosis.[1] Antibiotics should be started if there is worsening of symptoms or no improvement during the period of observation. Most clinical failures (84%) occur in the first 72 hours after the diagnosis of bacterial rhinosinusitis; consequently, if observation is indicated, it should be limited to 3 days.[18] If there is no improvement after 3 days, then antibiotics are indicated.

In a Cochrane Review of 6 placebo-controlled trials involving more than 600 patients who had symptoms of acute sinusitis for at least 7 days,[23] the use of antibiotics reduced the risk of treatment failure (relative risk 0.66, 95% confidence interval 0.44–0.98). However, in most randomized studies evaluating antibiotics for acute sinusitis, there is a significant response of patients in the placebo group. Although 90% of patients treated with antibiotics improve in 1 to 2 weeks, 80% of patients in the placebo arm show similar improvement. Thus, although the number needed to treat is 10 to improve 1 patient, physicians should keep in mind that many patients with acute sinusitis are better without antibiotic treatment.

Choice of Antibiotic for Acute Bacterial Sinusitis

Antibiotic therapy should be started immediately in those patients who meet clinical criteria for ABRS and with severe symptoms regardless of the duration.[18] Previously, amoxicillin was recommended as a first-line agent because of low cost and narrow spectrum. However, there is new evidence of increasing antimicrobial resistance to amoxicillin by the respiratory pathogens involved in ABRS. Amoxicillin-clavulanate improves coverage for these resistant pathogens. Local histograms for bacterial resistance should always be checked in order to understand local resistance trends. The IDSA 2012 guidelines are noted in **Table 3** and state[20]:

- Amoxicillin-clavulanate rather than amoxicillin alone is recommended as empirical antimicrobial therapy for adults who are not allergic to penicillin. The dose of amoxicillin-clavulanate for most patients would be either 500 mg/125 mg orally 3 times daily or 875 mg/125 mg orally twice daily.
- High-dose amoxicillin-clavulanate (2 g orally twice daily) is recommended in geographic areas with rates of penicillin-nonsusceptible *S pneumoniae* exceeding 10% and for patients who meet any of the following criteria: 65 years and older, recently hospitalized, treated with an antibiotic in the previous month, or immunocompromised.
- Doxycycline may be used as an alternative regimen for amoxicillin-clavulanate and can be used in patients with penicillin allergy. A respiratory fluoroquinolone (levofloxacin or moxifloxacin) is another option for penicillin-allergic patients.
- Macrolides (clarithromycin or azithromycin), trimethoprim-sulfamethoxazole, and second-generation or third-generation cephalosporins are not recommended

Table 3
Antibiotic recommendations for ABRS

First-line therapy	Amoxicillin-clavulanate 500 mg/125 mg 3 times a day or Amoxicillin-clavulanate 875 mg/125 mg twice a day
Penicillin allergy	Doxycycline 100 mg twice a day or Levofloxacin 500 mg daily or moxifloxacin 400 mg daily
High risk of penicillin-resistant *S pneumoniae*	Amoxicillin-clavulanate 2 g/125 mg twice a day
Pregnant and penicillin-allergic	Azithromycin 500 mg daily

for empirical therapy because of high rates of resistance of *S pneumoniae* (and of *H influenzae* for trimethoprim-sulfamethoxazole).
- Pregnant patients can be treated with amoxicillin-clavulanate (class B). If they are allergic to penicillin, use azithromycin (class B), because doxycycline (class D) and fluoroquinolones (class C) are contraindicated during pregnancy.

Duration of Antibiotic Therapy in Acute Bacterial Sinusitis

The IDSA guidelines recommend a 5-day to 7-day course of antibiotics (rather than 10–14 days) in adults. In a randomized trial using trimethoprim-sulfamethoxazole, researchers found that response rates were nearly identical with 3 days of antibiotics compared with 14 days.[21] In addition, other studies show that the adverse drug reaction rates are lower when 5 days of medicine are used compared with a 10-day course. Typically, patients have some response to antibiotic therapy after 3 to 5 days. However, age and comorbidities must be taken into account for a more prolonged response and may not show any improvement within 5 days of initiating antimicrobial therapy.[18]

Poor Response to Treatment or Recurrence

If the patient has symptoms that recur within 2 weeks of response to initial therapy, this may represent incomplete eradication of the pathogen. These patients with mild symptoms and a relapse should continue a longer course of the same antibiotic. However, if patients had only minimal response with the first-line therapy or relapse is more severe, this would require a change in the drug selected. These patients, who have worsening symptoms with initial empirical therapy or have a severe recurrence of symptoms, require treatment that offers a broader spectrum or a different class of antibiotic.

Second-line therapy from IDSA 2012 guidelines include:
- Amoxicillin-clavulanate 2000 mg/125 mg orally twice daily
- Levofloxacin 500 mg orally once daily
- Moxifloxacin 400 mg orally once daily

Treatment Considerations in Children with Sinusitis

In children with suspected sinusitis, there is a higher prevalence of β-lactamase producing *H influenzae* than in adults.[24] *S pneumoniae* has become less common in children. For this reason, amoxicillin-clavulanate is recommended for first-line treatment of sinusitis in children.

Although response rates to antibiotics in children with sinusitis are similar to adults, children treated with placebos have a markedly lower improvement rate compared with studies in adult populations. In 2 randomized controlled trials that used high-dose amoxicillin-clavulanate, patients in the treatment group had response rates of about 65% to 86%, whereas patients receiving placebo improved in only 35% to 40% of the time.[25–27] Based on one of these studies, the number needed to treat to result in 1 cure using high-dose amoxicillin-clavulanate is about 3, compared with 10 in adults.

Current recommendations are to use high-dose amoxicillin-clavulanate (90 mg/kg per day divided into 2 doses) in children less than 2 years of age, in children who are in day-care settings, those who have been hospitalized or treated with an antibiotic within the last 30 days and in localities in which penicillin resistance rates are more than 10%. Because of high rates of resistance, the use of macrolides or sulfamethoxazole is not recommended in children with sinusitis.

Chronic Sinusitis

In patients with chronic sinusitis, clinicians should consider referral to an otolaryngologist and treat potential underlying causes in order to lessen symptoms and reduce incidence of exacerbations. Nasal endoscopy is recommended in these patients to obtain middle meatal cultures in order to document persistent infection, determine presence of resistant pathogens, and direct further antibiotic coverage.[18] However, in most cases, antibiotics have not been shown to improve symptoms in either children or adults with chronic rhinosinusitis.[28,29] Conversely, a Cochrane review[30] found that intranasal corticosteroids improved symptom scores in patients with chronic rhinosinusitis without nasal polyps.

CT or nasal endoscopy can be used to evaluate masses or lesions noted on physical examination, patency of sinus passages, and anatomic variation. Multiple corrective surgical options are available and may be pursued by ear, nose, and throat specialists, often referred to as functional endoscopic sinus surgery (FESS), despite controversial evidence. A Cochrane review[31] found no clinically relevant difference in patients with chronic rhinosinusitis managed medically versus those who underwent FESS (either endoscopic middle meatal antrostomy or conventional inferior meatal antrostomy). However, in patients refractory to medical management, it remains a viable option, with some individual studies showing subjective improvement.[32–34]

COMPLICATIONS

If complicated disease is suspected by the symptoms, early referral is warranted. These patients may need urgent endoscopy, surgical biopsy, or additional diagnostic testing. A noncontrast CT scan of the sinuses may be ordered if the patient does not improve or symptoms worsen. This scan helps confirm that symptoms are a result of acute sinusitis and rule out other causes. If patients fail both first-line and second-line therapy, referral may be indicated for sinus cultures. The 2012 IDSA guidelines also have indications for less urgent specialty referral:

- Multiple recurrent episodes of ABRS (3–4 episodes per year), suggesting chronic rhinosinusitis
- Chronic rhinosinusitis (with or without polyps or asthma) with recurrent exacerbations of ABRS
- Patients with allergic rhinitis who need evaluation for possible immunotherapy

In these patients who are not responding to therapy, referral to an otolaryngologist is needed for cultures. These cultures are obtained by endoscopy from direct aspirate or endoscopy of the middle meatus and may be helpful to guide antimicrobial therapy, even when atypical pathogens are suspected.

However, more severe symptoms or comorbidities may necessitate more emergent referral. Symptoms indicating severe infection include high persistent fever, severe headache, orbital edema, visual changes, altered mental status, or meningeal signs. In these patients, fungal sinusitis or granulomatous disease must be considered. Acute fulminant invasive fungal rhinosinusitis may occur in patients who are immunosuppressed or who have poorly controlled diabetes. This disease is life threatening, and mortality is high despite therapy; emergent consultation with an otolaryngologist is required if suspected. Diagnosis is made by endoscopic examination and biopsy. Treatment of fungal sinusitis is surgical debridement and systemic antifungal therapy. Surgery may also be emergently indicated if there are other extrasinus complications of ABRS. Orbital abscess, meningitis, and brain abscess should also be considered in patients with severe symptoms.

PREVENTION

Primary prevention involves reducing the risk of an initial rhinosinusitis episode. Because most episodes of ABRS are preceded by a viral infection, prevention focuses on behaviors that decrease the risk of exposure to such pathogens. Patients can minimize exposure by proper hand hygiene, especially when in contact with others who are ill. Physicians can also advise patients of the increased risk of sinusitis associated with smoking.[35]

Secondary prevention applies to patients with chronic or recurrent ARS, either by minimizing symptoms or decreasing frequency of exacerbations. Nasal irrigation is recommended in these patients and after sinus surgery to improve mucociliary function, decrease edema, and remove colonizing pathogens through mechanical rinsing.[19,36–38] In these populations, physicians should consider additional factors, such as allergic rhinitis, immunocompromised state, and anatomic variation, which could alter management. Allergic rhinitis creates a hyperresponsive state, which may increase inflammation and cause edema, which can obstruct the paranasal sinuses and predispose patients to rhinosinusitis.[39] Immunodeficiencies should be suspected in patients with chronic or recurrent ARS associated with other upper respiratory infections, such as otitis media or pneumonia. Testing could include serum quantitative IgG, IgA, and IgM levels, as well as antibody responses to protein and polysaccharide antigens.[1]

Anatomic abnormalities that could obstruct the paranasal sinuses and trigger infection should also be considered. Indirect evidence for this idea is found in studies that show objective improvement in chronic rhinosinusitis after surgical correction of obstruction and anatomic abnormalities.[40,41]

GUIDELINES

Both the American Academy of Otolaryngology and the IDSA have published recommendations on the management of ABRS, which are consistent with the recommendations made here.[1,18] Diagnosis of ABRS should be differentiated from ARS caused by viral upper respiratory infections or other noninfectious causes by the presence of persistent symptoms beyond 10 days of onset, the presence of severe symptoms lasting 3 to 5 days, or the worsening of symptoms after an initial improvement (double sickening). Both panels recommend against use of imaging unless an alternative diagnosis or complication, such as orbital, intracranial, or soft tissue involvement, is suspected. However, radiographs may be obtained if the patient has modifying factors or comorbidities that predispose to complications. Complicated sinusitis should be evaluated with iodine contrast-enhanced CT or gadolinium-based MRI to detect involvement outside of the sinuses.

Antibiotic therapy should be initiated as soon as the clinical diagnosis of ABRS is made in order to shorten illness duration, provide symptomatic relief, and prevent complications. The approach of watchful waiting is indicated only if the diagnosis is uncertain. The IDSA recommends amoxicillin-clavulanate for empirical treatment in both children and adults.[18] In patients with a penicillin allergy, doxycycline or a respiratory fluoroquinolone is recommended because of high rates of S pneumoniae resistance with macrolides, oral cephalosporins, and trimethoprim-sulfamethoxazole.[18] Doxycycline is more cost effective than a respiratory fluoroquinolone but is not recommended in children because of teeth staining. High-dose antibiotic treatment is suggested in patients living in areas with more than 10% endemic rates of penicillin-resistant S pneumoniae, those with severe infection, day-care attendance, age younger than 2 or older than 65 years, recent hospitalization, antibiotic use within the preceding 4 to 6 weeks, or those who are immunocompromised. The recommended treatment duration is 5 to 7 days for adults and 10 to 14 days for children.

Patients may be treated symptomatically with oral or topical decongestants, although evidence for either is lacking. Oral decongestants theoretically can restore sinus patency; however, the effect is limited to the nasal cavity and does not continue into the paranasal sinuses. Topical decongestants provide more symptomatic relief but are limited to 3 days of use because of the risk of rebound congestion. Intranasal steroids can also be used as adjunctive therapy in patients with a history of allergic rhinitis to reduce the allergic response, thereby decreasing mucosal inflammation and permitting sinus drainage. Antihistamines are not recommended, because they may worsen congestion by producing a drying effect that is associated with slowed mucus transport.

Treatment failure is defined as symptom worsening or failure to improve after 3 to 5 days, at which time the physician should reassess the patient to confirm the diagnosis, consider antibiotic-resistant organisms, and detect complications. Physicians should also distinguish chronic or recurrent acute sinusitis from isolated episodes of acute bacterial sinusitis and assess patients with chronic or recurrent acute sinusitis for modifiable factors.

SUMMARY

Sinusitis affects 1 in 7 adults each year[1] and, even although it is common, controversy still exists regarding terminology, diagnostic criteria, indications for imaging, and treatment guidelines. Disease develops secondary to increased mucus production, decreased ciliary function, and subsequent obstruction of the ostiomeatal complex. Patients then present with symptoms of nasal congestion, purulent nasal discharge, and sinus tenderness suggestive of sinusitis.

Although most are caused by viral infections, acute bacterial sinusitis can be diagnosed when symptoms persist for longer than 10 days, or 3 to 5 days for severe symptoms, or worsen after a period of improvement. Typical offending organisms include S pneumoniae and H influenzae, but may include other respiratory pathogens, which should be considered based on the patient history and risk factors. Routine radiographic imaging is not recommended for diagnostic purposes and should be used only in cases of suspected complications.

Patients who are diagnosed with bacterial sinusitis should be started on amoxicillin-clavulanate, unless an allergy is reported, in which case, doxycycline or a respiratory fluoroquinolone is indicated, and treatment should be continued for 5 to 7 days in adults and 10 to 14 days in children.

Patients who fail to respond to antibiotic therapy should be suspected of having chronic sinusitis. These patients are more likely to have irreversible changes in their nasal and paranasal structures, which require additional therapy, including endoscopic surgery. Referral of these patients to an otolaryngologist for further evaluation is recommended. In addition, patients with suspected fungal sinusitis should be referred to an otolaryngologist acutely, because this condition has high mortality if not treated emergently.

REFERENCES

1. Rosenfeld RM, Andes D, Bhattacharyya N, et al. Clinical practice guideline: adult sinusitis. Otolaryngol Head Neck Surg 2007;137(Suppl):S1–31.
2. Weinberg EA, Brodsky L, Brody A, et al. Clinical classification as a guide to treatment of sinusitis in children. Laryngoscope 1997;107:241–6.

3. Evans KL. Diagnosis and management of sinusitis. Lancet 1994;309:1415–22.
4. Ohasi Y, Nakai Y. Reduced ciliary activity in chronic sinusitis. Acta Otolaryngol 1983;397(Suppl):3–9.
5. Ohasi Y, Nakai Y. Functional and morphological pathology of chronic sinusitis mucous membrane. Acta Otolaryngol Suppl 1983;397(Suppl):11–48.
6. Hueston WJ, Eberlein C, Johnson D, et al. Criteria used by clinicians to differentiate sinusitis from viral upper respiratory tract infection. J Fam Pract 1998;46: 487–92.
7. Little DR, Mann BL, Godbout CJ. How family physicians distinguish acute sinusitis from upper respiratory tract infection: a retrospective study. J Am Board Fam Pract 2000;13:101–6.
8. Adam P, Stiffman M, Blake RL Jr. A clinical trial of hypertonic saline nasal spray in subjects with the common cold or rhinosinusitis. Arch Fam Med 1998;7:39–43.
9. Williams JW, Simel DL. Does this patient have sinusitis? JAMA 1993;270:1242–6.
10. Lindbaeck M, Hjortdahl P, Johnsen UL. Use of symptoms, signs, and blood tests to diagnose acute sinusitis in primary care. J Fam Pract 1996;28:183–6.
11. Hansen JG, Schmidt H, Rosborg J, et al. Predicting acute maxillary sinusitis in a general practice population. BMJ 1995;311:233–6.
12. Gordts F, Clement PA, Buisseret T. Prevalence of sinusitis signs in a non-ENT population. ORL J Otorhinolaryngol Relat Spec 1996;58:315–9.
13. Henriksson G, Westrin JM, Kumlien J, et al. 13-year report on childhood sinusitis: clinical presentations, predisposing risk factors and possible means of prevention. Rhinology 1997;34:171–5.
14. Lanza DC, Kennedy DW. Adult rhinosinusitis defined. Otolaryngol Head Neck Surg 1997;117:S1–7.
15. Meltzer EO, Hamilos DL, Hadley JA, et al. Rhinosinusitis: establishing definitions for clinical research and patient care. Otolaryngol Head Neck Surg 2004;131: S1–62.
16. Wilson JF. In the clinic. Acute sinusitis. Ann Intern Med 2010;153:ITC31–5.
17. Young J, De Sutter A, Merenstein D, et al. Antibiotics for adults with clinically diagnosed acute rhinosinusitis: a meta-analysis of individual patient data. Lancet 2008;371:908.
18. Chow AW, Benninger MS, Brook I, et al. IDSA clinical practice guideline for acute bacterial rhinosinusitis in children and adults. Clin Infect Dis 2012;54:e1–72.
19. Fokkens W, Lund V, Bachert C, et al. EAACI position paper on rhinosinusitis and nasal polyps executive summary. Allergy 2005;60:583–601.
20. Hickner JM, Bartlett JG, Besser RE, et al. Principles of appropriate antibiotic use for acute rhinosinusitis in adults: background. Ann Intern Med 2001;134:498–505.
21. Williams JW Jr, Holleman DR Jr, Samsa GP, et al. Randomized controlled trial of 3 vs 10 days of trimethoprim/sulfamethoxazole for acute maxillary sinusitis. JAMA 1995;273:1015–21.
22. Williamson IG, Rumsby K, Benge S, et al. Antibiotics and topical nasal steroid for treatment of acute maxillary sinusitis: a randomized controlled trial. JAMA 2007; 298:2487–96.
23. Ahovuo-Saloranta A, Rautakorpi U-M, Borisenko OV, et al. Antibiotics for acute maxillary sinusitis. Cochrane Database Syst Rev 2008;(2):CD000243. http://dx.doi.org/10.1002/14651858.CD000243.pub2.
24. DeMuri GP, Wald ER. Acute bacterial sinusitis in children. N Engl J Med 2012;367: 1128–34.
25. Wald ER, Nash D, Eickhoof J. Effectiveness of amoxicillin-clavulanate potassium in the treatment of acute bacterial sinusitis in children. Pediatrics 2009;124:9–15.

26. Wald ER, Chiponis D, Ledesma-Medina J. Comparative effectiveness of amoxicillin and amoxicillin-clavulanate potassium in acute paranasal sinus infections in children: a double-blind, placebo-controlled trial. Pediatrics 1986;77:795–800.
27. Berger G, Steinberg DM, Popovtzer A, et al. Endoscopy versus radiography for the diagnosis of acute bacterial rhinosinusitis. Eur Arch Otorhinolaryngol 2005; 262:416–22.
28. Piromchai P, Thanaviratananich S, Laopaiboon M. Systemic antibiotics for chronic rhinosinusitis without nasal polyps in adults. Cochrane Database Syst Rev 2011;(5):CD008233.
29. Duiker SS, Parker S, Hensel WA. Clinical inquiries. Do antibiotics improve outcomes in chronic rhinosinusitis? J Fam Pract 2004;53(3):237–40.
30. Snidvongs K, Kalish L, Sacks R, et al. Topical steroid for chronic rhinosinusitis without polyps. Cochrane Database Syst Rev 2011;(8):CD009274.
31. Khalil HS, Nunez DA. Functional endoscopic sinus surgery for chronic rhinosinusitis. Cochrane Database Syst Rev 2006;(3):CD004458.
32. Senior BA, Kennedy DW, Tanabodee J, et al. Long-term results of functional endoscopic sinus surgery. Laryngoscope 1998;108(2):151–7.
33. Lund VJ, Mackay IS. Outcome assessment of endoscopic sinus surgery. J R Soc Med 1994;87:70–2.
34. Lund VJ, Scadding GK. Objective assessment of endoscopic sinus surgery in the management of chronic rhinosinusitis: an update. J Laryngol Otol 1994;108: 749–53.
35. Lieu JE, Feinstein AR. Confirmations and surprises in the association of tobacco use with sinusitis. Arch Otolaryngol Head Neck Surg 2000;126:940–6.
36. Slavin RG, Spector SL, Bernstein IL, et al. The diagnosis and management of sinusitis: a practice parameter update. J Allergy Clin Immunol 2005;116(Suppl 6): S13–47.
37. Benninger MS, Anon J, Mabry RL. The medical management of rhinosinusitis. Otolaryngol Head Neck Surg 1997;117(Suppl):S41–9.
38. Friedman M, Vidyasagar R, Joseph N. A randomized, prospective, double-blind study on the efficacy of dead sea salt nasal irrigations. Laryngoscope 2006;116: 878–82.
39. Alho OP, Karttunen R, Karttunen TJ. Nasal mucosa in the natural colds: effects of allergic rhinitis and susceptibility to recurrent sinusitis. Clin Exp Immunol 2004; 137:366–72.
40. Senior BA, Kennedy DW. Management of sinusitis in the asthmatic patient. Ann Allergy Asthma Immunol 1996;77:6–15.
41. Sipila J, Antila J, Suonpaa J. Pre- and postoperative evaluation of patients with nasal obstruction undergoing endoscopic sinus surgery. Eur Arch Otorhinolaryngol 1996;253:237–9.

Epistaxis: Evaluation and Treatment

Daniel J. Morgan, MD[a,b,*], Rick Kellerman, MD[b]

KEYWORDS

- Epistaxis • Uncontrolled nosebleed • Family physician

KEY POINTS

- Epistaxis, or nosebleed, is a common disorder that many patients will experience.
- Most patients go to the emergency room when they have an uncontrolled nosebleed, but they may present to an outpatient office.
- Most nosebleeds are not life-threatening and can be managed conservatively.
- Occasionally, hospital admission, referral to an otolaryngologist physician, and/or blood transfusion may be necessary.

EPIDEMIOLOGY

Although epistaxis can occur at any age, there is a bimodal distribution of children up to age 10 and adults greater than age 50.[1]

The lifetime prevalence of epistaxis is about 60% in the general population. Ten percent will present to a physician, and only a few are ever seen by an otorhinolaryngologist.[1-3] Individuals older than age 50 represent 40% of those requiring medical attention and tend to have more serious bleeds. Children younger than 10 years of age with a nosebleed tend to have an uncomplicated course because their nosebleeds are usually from the anterior nasal blood supply and require limited intervention.[4] Children under the age of 2 with nosebleeds are rare and warrant consideration of trauma (accidental and nonaccidental), nasal foreign body, and/or a systemic medical condition (bleeding disorder).[5]

Thirty-three percent of all emergent admissions for ear, nose, and throat problems are for epistaxis. The median age for hospital admission for epistaxis is 70.[6]

ANATOMY

Nosebleeds from the anterior nasal blood supply are more common than bleeds from the posterior blood supply. In fact, 90% of nosebleeds are from the anterior nasal

Disclosures Funding Sources: None.
Conflicts of Interest: None.
[a] Wesley Medical Center, Wichita, KS, USA; [b] Department of Family and Community Medicine, University of Kansas School of Medicine-Wichita, 1010 North Kansas, Wichita, KS 67214, USA
* Corresponding author.
E-mail address: danthemedicineman5162010@gmail.com

blood supply.[7] Most of these occur in the Little's area, where the Kieselbach plexus of blood vessels is located (**Fig. 1**). The Kieselbach plexus is made up of the septal branch of the superior labial artery, the septal branch of the anterior ethmoid artery, and the nasal branch of the anterior ethmoid artery.

Posterior bleeds are much more difficult to evaluate and treat because the posterior nares blood supply is more difficult to access than the anterior nares blood supply. The posterior nasal area is supplied by the posteriolateral branches of the sphenopalatine artery. In rare situations, posterior nosebleeds are due to a malignancy, internal carotid aneurysm, or major trauma (see **Fig. 1**).

CAUSE

There are several possible causes of nosebleeds that will commonly be seen by primary care physicians. The most common is trauma from nose picking. The Kieselbach plexus is just inside the opening of the nares and can easily be exposed by excoriation. Nose bleeds from blunt trauma due to a motor vehicle collision or physical altercation is usually from an anterior source. Sinusitis may be associated with bleeding from the nose.

In children, insertion of a foreign body may cause a traumatic nosebleed. The patient or an adult trying to remove the object may inflict traumatic bleeding. If the object has been in place for longer than 24 hours, the bleeding may be accompanied by purulent nasal drainage. Foreign bodies are usually located in the inferior nasal turbinate.[8]

Dry air from the outside environment or from a centrally heated building can result in mucosa that is easily irritated and may bleed with little provocation. Inflammation from viral or allergic rhinitis may cause the nasal mucosa to become friable. Because the nasal turbinates may swell due to underlying allergy or infection, the mucosa may bleed easily and profusely.

One treatment of allergic rhinitis is topical steroids. Topical steroids themselves have been shown to increase the risk of nosebleeds, so consideration must be given to the treatment of nasal allergy symptoms in a patient with a history of nosebleeds.[9]

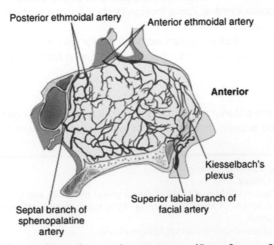

Fig. 1. Blood vessels supplying the nasal passageway. (*From* Savage S. Management of epistaxis. In: Pfenninger JL, Fowler GC, editors. Pfenninger and Fowler's procedures for primary care. 3rd edition. Philadelphia: Saunders; 2011; with permission.)

Septal deviation or perforation may present as a nosebleed. These anatomic anomalies of the septum may be from trauma, past surgery, or drug use (ie, cocaine). Nosebleeds in a patient with a septal perforation can be difficult to evaluate because patients may have bleeding from both nostrils.

If nosebleeds are recurrent or difficult to control, the primary care physician should consider that the cause may be from a rarely encountered disorder (**Box 1**). Aneurysms, vascular malformations, and sinus tumors may present as bleeding from the nose.

PREVENTION

There are few large studies on epistaxis prevention, but experts indicate that liberal application of petroleum jelly to each nostril to prevent mucosal drying is an efficacious and cost-effective way to prevent anterior epistaxis. Several small studies have shown that antiseptic cream for recurrent epistaxis in children is effective.[10] It is speculated to be beneficial in adults as well. A humidification unit, especially in dry climates and in centrally heated areas, should be used while sleeping, especially after having a nosebleed. Parents should keep children's fingernails trimmed to minimize trauma from nose picking.

Box 1
Conditions associated with epistaxis

Vascular malformation/telangiectasia

- Osler-Weber-Rendu syndrome
- Angioma
- Aneurysm of the carotid artery

Neoplasm

- Squamous cell carcinoma
- Adenoid cystic carcinoma
- Melanoma
- Inverted papilloma (these tend to be more common in patients of Asian heritage)[7]

Coagulopathy (primary or iatrogenic)

- Thrombocytopenia
- von Willebrand disease
- Hemophilia
- Liver disease
- Leukemia
- HIV

Barotrauma

Medications

- Nasal steroids
- Cocaine
- Anticoagulation (Warfarin, clopidogrel)
- Chronic use of nasal vasoconstrictors

EVALUATION

When first examining a patient with epistaxis, the clinician should focus on determining if the patient has a patent airway and cardiovascular stability. If the patient has severe bleeding and/or hypotension, intravenous fluid boluses, a complete blood count, and type and cross match for blood transfusion will be necessary.

At times, patients will have bleeding from both nostrils. The clinician should ask on which side the bleeding started. To assess severity, the clinician should try to determine when the bleeding started, how much blood has been lost (to the patient's best approximation), and if the bleeding is a chronic or recurrent problem. Symptoms of hematemesis or hemoptysis may indicate a posterior bleed, which tends to be more voluminous than anterior bleeds, or a large anterior bleed. A complete past medical history should be taken, focusing on conditions that could make a nosebleed worse or more likely, such as a history of head and neck tumors, medications or drugs (anticoagulants, intranasal cocaine, intranasal steroids), primary coagulopathy, trauma, previous or recent nasal or sinus surgeries, and HIV (because of platelet dysfunction or thrombocytopenia). Blood loss from nosebleeds may complicate existing heart and lung disease, so asking about dyspnea, sweating, chest pain/pressure, left arm pain, jaw pain, and syncope is important.

It was previously thought that nonsteroidal anti-inflammatory drugs, aspirin, and high blood pressure were causes of nosebleeds. There is no association between nonsteroidal anti-inflammatory drugs and epistaxis. Aspirin has been shown in some studies to increase the risk of epistaxis and in other studies there is no difference compared with nonaspirin users.[11,12] Most of the aspirin studies are retrospective, however, so conclusive evidence is lacking. A population-based study has shown that there is no association between hypertension and epistaxis.[13]

Before performing a physical examination, the clinician should wear appropriate personal protection equipment including goggles, a gown, gloves, and a facemask. It should be determined on which side the bleed is occurring, which can usually be determined from the history. However, occasionally patients will have bilateral bleeding or cannot give an accurate history, so close examination with a nasal speculum may be necessary. If a more extensive examination is indicated, placing a pledget moistened with a vasoconstrictive medication (eg, oxymetazoline) and an anesthetic (2% lidocaine) may be required. After several minutes, the pledget can be removed and visualization will be improved (**Fig. 2**).

Once the patient is anesthetized, they should lie back at 30°. Good lighting should be available. Using a nasal specula, the anterior mucosa is examined, focusing on the Kiesselbach plexus, which is located in the Little's area (see **Fig. 1**). Blood clots may obscure optimal visualization and having the patient blow their nose to remove clots will help clear the nares. A small suction catheter can also be used to remove clots.

Laboratory workup is typically not indicated unless the bleeding is profuse or the patient suffers complications. If the patient is anti-coagulated, testing the international normalized ratio is justified. If the patient is hemodynamically unstable, then a complete blood count, basic metabolic panel, international normalized ratio and other coagulation studies, and a type and cross match for potential blood transfusion are required. Vital signs may need to be monitored frequently.

Epistaxis is relatively common among patients who are medically anticoagulated, though treatment rarely requires anticoagulant reversal.[14] Patients who are on warfarin and in the therapeutic range for their condition will not require anticoagulation reversal if hemostasis is achieved.

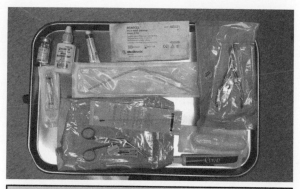

Items for an epistaxis tray
Nasal decongestant
Local anesthetic
Silver nitrate sticks or electric cautery
Bayonet forceps
Nasal speculum
Frazier suction with appropriate tip
Posterior bleed balloon (ie, Epistat and Storz T-3100)
Packing materials, such as pledgets or preformed packing materials, such as Pope Epistaxis Packing (Medtronic ENT, Medtronic USA Inc, Jacksonville, FL, USA) and Rapid Rhino (Arthrocare ENT, Sunnyvale, CA, USA)

Fig. 2. Epistaxis tray.

DIFFERENTIATING BETWEEN ANTERIOR NASAL BLEEDS AND POSTERIOR NASAL BLEEDS

Determining an anterior nasal bleed from a posterior nasal bleed is important and can be difficult. Posterior nasal bleeds tend to bleed more heavily than anterior nasal bleeds, although anterior ones can bleed heavily on occasion. A nosebleed with a large volume of blood does not necessarily mean it is from a posterior source. However, a small bleed usually indicates an anterior source. The patient who has bilateral bleeding may have a posterior nasal source. If the side from which the bleeding originates cannot be determined from the history and initial examination, bilateral anterior nasal packing can be placed. If the patient is still having heavy bleeding after bilateral anterior nasal packing, then a posterior source is more likely.

Bilateral bleeding may also occur if the patient has a nasal septal defect or bilateral nasal lesions.

TREATMENT FOR ANTERIOR NOSEBLEEDS

While performing the history, the patient should sit and lean forward to keep blood from running into the posterior pharynx. Then oxymetazoline (Afrin) should be sprayed twice into the bleeding side. The patient should be instructed to continuously hold pressure on the nares by pinching the nostrils tightly (**Fig. 3**), for 10 to 15 minutes, giving the clinician enough time to take the history. A small retrospective study showed

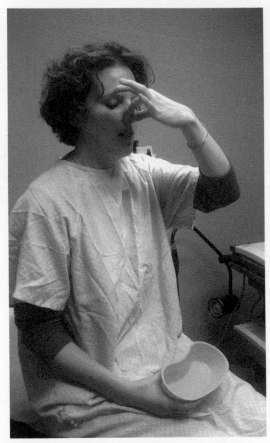

Fig. 3. Patient positioned and pinching nostrils tightly for treatment of minor epistaxis.

that 65% of emergency room patients with epistaxis were successfully treated with oxymetazoline (Afrin) and continuous pressure.[15]

Anterior nosebleeds can often be located visually without much difficulty and direct treatment can be undertaken. The 2 most common direct treatments are chemical cautery (eg, silver nitrate) and electrocautery. Complications include septal perforation, infection, rhinorrhea, and worsening bleeding. Chemical and electrocautery are equally effective and have about the same complication rate.[16] Direct treatment is ideal for the patient's comfort because this avoids uncomfortable nasal packing. If there is any rebleeding or the clinician cannot find the source, nasal packing may be necessary.

The patient should don a gown and hold an emesis basin to catch any bleeding. Before the examination, a vasoconstrictor (eg, oxymetazoline) and anesthetic (eg, Lidocaine 2%) should be applied. The vasoconstrictor will reduce bleeding in the affected area and improve visualization while the anesthetic will make the procedure more comfortable for the patient.

If the bleeding area cannot be visualized because of clots, they should be removed. Large clots may be removed manually with suction or forceps. If this is not desired or successful, the patient may blow their nose to remove the clots. The size of clots removed may be significant. At times, the bleeding will stop from simply removing the clots. Clots may need to be removed before any vasoconstrictive medications will be effective. If the medication has already been applied, then the physician should consider reapplication, because the clots may have been covering the mucosa, preventing the medication from absorbing into the tissue.

If the bleeding continues after applying direct pressure and removing any clots, an option is to apply a pledget or cotton ball soaked with a decongestant on the side of the nose that is bleeding. If the bleeding source location is identified, the cotton ball or pledget should be placed directly on the bleeding area. However, if the bleeding source's location is not visualized, then the pledget may have to be placed blindly. In that case, a pledget should be placed in the 3 most likely sites of an anterior bleed: one superior, one posterior, and one inferior. The pledgets should stay in place for the next 10 minutes.

When the pledget is removed, the bleeding source will usually be identified by an erosion on the mucosa or a small locus of bleeding. A small amount of silver nitrate or electrocautery can be applied. Spot application may be all that is required. In some cases, wider application may be necessary. One technique that works well is to surround the bleeding vessel in a circular motion, cauterizing the surrounding mucosa and slowly moving toward the center of the spiral, eventually cauterizing the bleeding vessel.[17]

After making sure that the bleeding has stopped, a small amount of ointment or petroleum jelly should be applied to keep the area moist. It may be prudent to monitor the patient for the next 30 minutes to make sure the nose does not start bleeding again.

If the above measures do not stop the bleeding, an anterior pack will need to be inserted and remain in place for 24 to 48 hours. Packing made specifically for nosebleeds is available (Pope Epistaxis Packing and Rapid Rhino). Packing made specifically for nosebleeds is desired because of the faster speed of insertion, lower amount of trauma, and increased effectiveness than traditional methods. Each type of packing will have specific instructions on their use. In general, preformed packing products are covered with a lubricant and inserted quickly but gently into the affected side. The packing usually expands by absorbing the blood that is present. If the packing does not expand, irrigating with 5 to 10 mL of saline may be necessary. The costs of these products are in the range of 100 to 150 dollars (US).

If these products are not available, an anterior pack can be fashioned from xeroform petrolatum gauze or from 4 to 6 feet of $\frac{1}{2}$-inch gauze coated with antibiotic ointment or petroleum jelly. Different methods for insertion are possible. One method starts by inserting the free end of the gauze into the affected nares as far posteriorly as possible without entering the pharynx.[1] An alternative method involves folding the gauze in half, making it 2 to 3 feet in length, and then inserting the folded pleat first.[18] Whichever method is used, the inserted gauze will need to be pressed down firmly against the inferior nares. Subsequent rows of gauze are inserted and pressed down firmly. This process will be repeated, in an accordion-like fashion, until the nose is packed completely (**Figs. 4** and **5**).

If the anterior packing decreases the amount of bleeding, but does not stop it entirely, then placing another pack on the unaffected side can increase the amount of intranasal pressure and may stop the bleeding.

After placing the packing, the physician will need to monitor the patient for 30 minutes to observe for any possible posterior bleeding. If there is no bleeding, the physician may discharge the patient home. The patient should be sent home with prophylactic antibiotics that will cover for nasal pathogens. First-line treatment is cephalexin 250 mg 4 times a day or amoxicillin/clavulanate 250 mg 3 times a day.

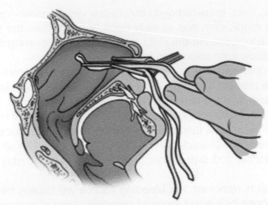

Fig. 4. Start the packing on the inferior turbinate. (*From* Savage S. Management of epistaxis. In: Pfenninger JL, Fowler GC, editors. Pfenninger and Fowler's procedures for primary care. 3rd edition. Philadelphia: Saunders; 2011; with permission.)

For a penicillin allergy, clindamycin 150 mg 4 times a day or trimethoprim/sulfameth-oxazole DS twice a day is appropriate. The patient will need follow-up in 24 to 48 hours, at which point the anterior pack will be removed. If the patient has bleeding, fever, drainage, or increased pain, they should return sooner than 48 hours for evaluation. Before removing the packing, irrigating the packing with 5 to 10 mL of saline and waiting 5 to 10 minutes will help keep the gauze from sticking to the mucosa during removal.

The patient should avoid picking or blowing their nose for at least a week. Bending over or straining may increase the risk of a recurrent bleed.

TREATMENT FOR POSTERIOR NOSEBLEEDS

The patient with a posterior nasal bleed can be difficult to treat in the emergency room or the office. If anterior packing has been placed, but the patient is suspected to have

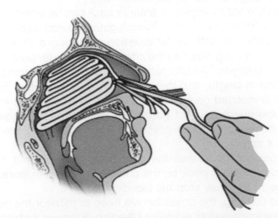

Fig. 5. Continue packing in accordion-like fashion until nasal passageway is completely full of gauze. (*From* Savage S. Management of epistaxis. In: Pfenninger JL, Fowler GC, editors. Pfenninger and Fowler's procedures for primary care. 3rd edition. Philadelphia: Saunders; 2011; with permission.)

a posterior nasal bleed, the anterior packing will need to be removed. The patient will need to be reanesthetized.

Several posterior balloon packs are available and effective (ie, Epistat and Storz T-3100). The balloon should be lubricated with a water-soluble lubricant. The device should be inserted into the nasal passageway of the affected side, until it can be visualized in the oropharynx. The balloon is then inflated with 7 to 10 mL saline. Next, the balloon is pulled firmly, but not aggressively, back into the nasal cavity. An umbilical clamp or equivalent device is placed on the nasal end of the tube to prevent movement of the balloon. A piece of gauze can be placed between the clamp and the nares to prevent compression necrosis. If the balloon is overinflated, or not properly placed, tissue necrosis of the posterior nasal cavity can occur.

In some offices and emergency rooms, a special balloon may not be available, and a Foley catheter may be used as a substitute. A small-diameter (10–14 Fr) catheter should be used to make the placement more comfortable. Clipping off the hard end of the catheter distal to the balloon will help prevent abrasive rubbing of the posterior pharynx. The device should be inserted in a manner similar to the specialty device. The well-lubricated Foley catheter should be inserted into the affected side until it can be visualized in the oropharynx. Then, approximately 10 mL normal saline should be infused into the Foley catheter balloon. The catheter should be retracted until the balloon is seated in the posterior nasal cavity. An umbilical clamp or equivalent device should then be placed on the portion of the catheter outside the nose to prevent the Foley balloon from moving. A small amount of gauze can be placed between the clamp and the nares to prevent tissue necrosis (**Fig. 6**).[1]

Some nasal bleeds may have an anterior and posterior component, especially in cases that are secondary to underlying pathologic abnormality (ie, Osler-Weber-Rendu syndrome). In these cases, the posterior nasal packing should be placed, using the technique described above. Then, if an anterior bleed is also suspected, placement of an anterior pack may be necessary. While placing the anterior packing, the physician must make sure to hold some tension on the catheter to make sure it stays

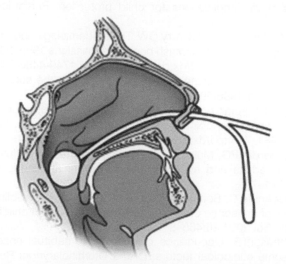

Fig. 6. The posterior balloon should be seated firmly in the posterior pharynx. (*From* Savage S. Management of epistaxis. In: Pfenninger JL, Fowler GC, editors. Pfenninger and Fowler's procedures for primary care. 3rd edition. Philadelphia: Saunders; 2011; with permission.)

in place. After placing the anterior packing, the physician will attempt to visualize the balloon in the oropharynx to make sure it is still placed properly. Placing the anterior packing can push the posterior balloon too inferior to be effective. The balloon must be repositioned by gently pulling on the catheter, making sure to avoid dislodging the anterior packing.

The patient with posterior packing will need to be admitted for close monitoring. The patient will require prophylactic antibiotics while the foreign body is in place. To prevent tissue necrosis and infection, the packing will need to be removed within 48 to 72 hours.

A potential complication of both anterior and posterior packing that is kept in place for extended periods of time is toxic shock syndrome.

The risk of rebleeding and complicated bleeds from posterior nasal bleeds may require otorhinolaryngology consultation. Even when appropriate measures are taken to control a posterior nasal bleed, 25% will not stop.[18] An ear, nose, and throat specialist may perform endoscopic surgery to ligate the sphenopalatine or anterior ethmoid artery. Angiographic embolization can also be performed by interventional radiology.

REFERENCES

1. Kucik CJ, Clenney T. Management of epistaxis. Am Fam Physician 2005;71(2): 305–11.
2. Melia L, McGarry GW. Epistaxis: update on management. Curr Opin Otolaryngol Head Neck Surg 2011;19:30–5.
3. Tomkinson A, Roblin DG, Flanagan P, et al. Patterns of hospital attendance with epistaxis. Rhinology 1997;35(3):129–31.
4. Brown N, Berkowitz R. Epistaxis in healthy children requiring hospital admission. Int J Pediatr Otorhinolaryngol 2004;68(9):1181–4.
5. McIntosh N, Mok JY, Margerison A. Epidemiology of oronasal hemorrhage in the first 2 years of life: implications for child protection. Pediatrics 2007;120(5): 1074–8.
6. Walker TW, Macfarlane TV, McGarry GW. The epidemiology and chronobiology of epistaxis: an investigation of Scottish hospital admissions 1995–2004. Clin Otolaryngol 2007;32(5):361–5. http://dx.doi.org/10.1111/j.1749-4486.2007.01530.
7. Alvi A, Joyner-Triplett N. Acute epistaxis. How to spot the source and stop the flow. Postgrad Med 1996;99(5):94–6.
8. Kalan A, Tariq M. Foreign bodies in the nasal cavities: a comprehensive review of the aetiology, diagnostic pointers, and therapeutic measures. Postgrad Med J 2000;76(898):484–7. http://dx.doi.org/10.1136/pmj.76.898.484.
9. Rosenblut A, Bardin PG, Muller B, et al. Long-term safety of fluticasone furoate nasal spray in adults and adolescents with perennial allergic rhinitis. Allergy 2007;62(9):1071–7.
10. Kubba H, MacAndie C, Botma M, et al. A prospective, single-blind, randomized controlled trial of antiseptic cream for recurrent epistaxis in childhood. Clin Otolaryngol Allied Sci 2001;26:465–8.
11. Beran M, Petruson B. Occurrence of epistaxis in habitual nose-bleeders and analysis of some etiological factors. ORL J Otorhinolaryngol Relat Spec 1986; 48(5):297–303.
12. Tay HL, Evans JM, McMahon AD, et al. Aspirin, nonsteroidal anti-inflammatory drugs, and epistaxis. A regional record linkage case control study. Ann Otol Rhinol Laryngol 1998;107(8):671–4.

13. Flavio D, Fuchs FD, Moreira LB, et al. Absence of association between hypertension and epistaxis: a population-based study. Blood Press 2003;12:145–8.
14. Nitu IC, Perry DJ, Lee CA. Clinical experience with the use of clotting factor concentrates in oral anticoagulation reversal. Clin Lab Haematol 1998;20(6):363–7.
15. Krempl GA, Noorily AD. Use of oxymetazoline in the management of epistaxis. Ann Otol Rhinol Laryngol 1995;104(9 Pt 1):704–6.
16. Toner JG, Walby AP. Comparison of electro and chemical cautery in the treatment of anterior epistaxis. J Laryngol Otol 1990;104(8):617–8.
17. Riviello RJ. Otolaryngologic procedures. In: Roberts JR, Hedges JR, editors. Clinical procedures in emergency medicine. 4th edition. Philadelphia: WB Saunders; 2004. p. 1300.
18. Beck R, Hizon JW. Management of epistaxis. From Pfenninger and Fowler's procedures for primary care. 2nd edition. St Louis (MO): Mosby; 2003. p. 465–73.

Diseases of the Mouth

Hugh Silk, MD, MPH

KEYWORDS

- Oral • Stomatitis • Candidiasis • Caries • Oral cancers • Leukoplakia

KEY POINTS

- The most common infection and disease of the mouth is caries. Caries is a chronic, transmissible disease caused by bacteria using sugar to create an acidic environment that erodes the teeth.
- Candidiasis is an infection of the oral mucosa by the Candida species. The most prominent candida infection in humans is *Candida albicans*.
- Approximately 50% of children will have some form of gingivitis; for adults, it is as much as 90% when all types and causes are included. Gingivitis is very prevalent during pregnancy due to hormonal changes.
- Benign bony protuberances arise from the cortical plate and consist of lamellar bone. They are more common in the hard palate of the mouth but can also occur in the floor of the mouth. They are likely congenital but do not develop until adulthood.
- Clinicians should pay close attention to a history of nonhealing ulcer or mass in the mouth or on the lip, or any area that bleeds easily or has unexplained pain. Other concerning symptoms for oral cancer may include dysphagia/odynophagia, chronic sore throat or hoarseness, or unexplained ear pain.

INTRODUCTION

The mouth is the gateway to the body.[1] Disease in the mouth can cause systemic diseases (eg, bacterial endocarditis), and systemic disease can also lead to complications in the mouth (eg, Behcet disease). Patients often present first to their primary care provider with oral symptoms. Medical clinicians often defer diseases of the mouth to dental professionals, oral surgeons, and otolaryngologists; however, medical professionals should be comfortable with the diagnosis and initial management of many common diseases of the oral cavity. This article discusses 3 major categories of disease within the mouth (excluding the tongue and salivary glands):

1. Mouth infections (caries and complications, candidiasis)
2. Inflammatory conditions (gingivitis, periodontitis, and stomatitis)
3. Common benign and malignant lesions (bony tori, mucocele, lichen planus, leukoplakia, cancer).

Department of Family Medicine and Community Health, University of Massachusetts Medical School, Worcester, MA, USA
E-mail address: hugh.silk@umassmed.edu

Prim Care Clin Office Pract 41 (2014) 75–90
http://dx.doi.org/10.1016/j.pop.2013.10.011 **primarycare.theclinics.com**
0095-4543/14/$ – see front matter © 2014 Elsevier Inc. All rights reserved.

INFECTIONS OF THE MOUTH
Caries

Description
The most common infection and disease of the mouth is caries. Caries is a chronic, transmissible disease caused by bacteria using sugar to create an acidic environment that erodes the teeth. Over time this process leads to holes (cavities) in the tooth's structure. The predominant bacterium involved is *Streptococcus mutans,* although the disease may have more to do with a disruption of a complex biofilm on the teeth than the overpopulation of one species. Fluoride and saliva are protective factors.[2]

Risk factors
Risks for caries are multifactorial, including physical and socioeconomic factors. See **Box 1**.

Prevalence
Nearly 24% of adults aged 20 to 64 have untreated dental caries and 84% have had a dental restoration.[3] The western developed countries tend to have more caries compared with lesser developed countries and this is thought to be second to the predominance of concentrated refined sweets in many countries.

Clinical implications
Untreated caries can lead to local and systemic infections. A cavity invades the pulp and root of the tooth, which includes the nerves and blood supply. This local infection can spread through surrounding gingival tissue, form an abscess, penetrate other layers of anatomy such as the cheek or airway, and ultimately infect the meninges or bloodstream. At a minimum, untreated cavities can cause pain and at worst has caused death through meningitis.

Diagnostic options and dilemmas
Routine screening examinations by medical and dental professionals can help identify caries early. Most professional organizations recommend an examination every 6 months. Mouth radiographs done periodically (common recommendation is every 2 years) can also help diagnose disease in the early stages.

Box 1
Risk factors for caries in adults

Previous caries

High oral bacterial counts (mainly *S mutans*)

Inadequate oral hygiene (brushing with fluoridated toothpaste and flossing)

Inadequate exposure to fluoride

Frequent consumption of sugary foods, snacks, and drinks

Low socioeconomic status

Physical or mental disabilities (making it difficult to brush/floss)

Existing appliances (trapping food)

Decreased salivary flow (due to medications or disease states)

Exposed roots (in elderly due to lack of enamel on roots)

Management

Prevention is the key. The patient should be advised to brush teeth twice daily with fluoridated toothpaste and floss daily.[4] An oscillating toothbrush is more effective than a regular toothbrush for preventing oral disease in adults.[5] Routine screening is suggested as above. Children and adolescents should also be considered for fluoride varnish treatments, supplemental fluoride if primary water supply is not fluoridated, and sealants of secondary molars. Early caries can be treated with restoration; deeper cavities will require root canal or extractions.[1] Secondary infections require antibiotics, incision and drainage, and definitive treatment of the tooth with restoration or extraction.[6] A delay in treatment can lead to spread of infection as outlined above. Initial antibiotics include penicillin (loading dose of 1000 mg, followed by 500 mg 3–4 times daily for 7–10 days) but broader antibiotics (such as clindamycin; loading dose of 600 mg, followed by 300 mg orally 3 times daily for 7–10 days) should be used if infection is spreading.[7] Secondary infections (cellulitis, meningitis) require hospitalization with intravenous antibiotics, computed tomographic imaging,[8] and consultation. Pain should be managed with acetaminophen and ibuprofen; depending on the degree of infection and pain, a short course of opioids may be necessary.[9]

Candidiasis

Description

Candidiasis is an infection of the oral mucosa by candida species. The most prominent candida infection in humans is *Candida albicans* (**Fig. 1**).

Risk factors

Candida species are normal inhabitants of the gastrointestinal tract. Those that are immunocompromised are more susceptible to oral candidal infections, including elderly, infants, HIV-positive individuals, patients with cancer, and diabetes or those with glucose intolerance.[10] Certain medications cause individuals to be more prone, including antibacterial therapy (especially broad-spectrum antibiotics, which disrupt normal protective flora), inhaled steroids,[11] and chemotherapy. Dentures also can get infected with Candida and the surrounding area may only be erythematous and not white.

Prevalence

Candidiasis is not common in the general public; annual estimates are 50 in 100,000. However, in high-risk populations the numbers are more prevalent: 5% to 7% of

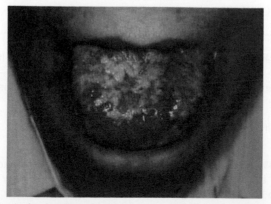

Fig. 1. Oral candidiasis. (*From* López-Martínez R. Candidosis, a new challenge. Clin Dermatol 2010;28(2):178–84; with permission.)

babies less than 1 month old; 9% to 31% of AIDS patients; nearly 20% of patients with cancer.[12]

Clinical implications

The diagnosis for candidiasis is usually made through a history of risk factors and symptoms (including painless white patches in the mouth). Physical examination of white patches confirms the diagnosis. The white layer can be partially wiped off and there can be an erythematous mucosa underlying. Complications include a descending spread of the infection along the gastrointestinal tract causing esophageal and gastric candidiasis. Candida of the mouth can also present solely as angular cheilitis at the corners of the mouth, resulting in cracks in the skin. Candidiasis of dentures may present as only erythema of the mucosa.

Diagnostic options and dilemmas

Diagnosis can be aided with a slide preparation looking for hyphae. If pH is checked, it should be less than 4.5. If there is any doubt of a diagnosis, a culture can be obtained. A culture can also be helpful for recalcitrant infection to confirm species and sensitivities. Differential diagnosis includes leukoplakia, lichen planus, geographic tongue, and milk or other white foods.

Management

Prevention includes modifying risk factors (avoid antibiotics, use narrow spectrum antibiotics, consider probiotics when using antibiotics, rinse after inhaled steroid use). For treatment, Nystatin suspension, 100,000 U/mL given 4 to 6 times daily, is a common, effective treatment. It also comes as a pastille.[13] Clotrimazole (Mycelex), 10 mg troche, sucked on 20 minutes 5 times a day for 7 to 14 days is an alternative. For angular cheilitis, Nystatin ointment can be prescribed: 100,000 U/g to corners of mouth 2 to 3 times daily for 3 weeks. If dentures are involved, proper cleaning is important[14]; one technique is to clean with diluted (1:20) bleach. For infants with thrush, be sure to boil all pacifiers and bottle nipples. Infants should be treated with nystatin suspension 0.5 mL in each cheek 4 times daily until better, which is usually 7 to 10 days. Mother's breasts should be treated as needed in breastfed babies with topical antifungals such as nystatin to the nipples of the breasts for the same duration. Oral agents (fluconazole or equivalent) can be used as second-line treatment or in cases of esophageal candidiasis.

INFLAMMATORY CONDITIONS OF THE MOUTH
Gingivitis

Description

Gingivitis is a reversible form of inflammation of the gingival (**Fig. 2**). It is a mild form of periodontal disease. Classifications include plaque-induced, non-plaque-induced, and then gingivitis secondary to medications and systemic diseases.[15]

Risk factors

Risk factors for gingivitis are multifactorial. See **Box 2**.

Prevalence

Approximately 50% of children will have some form of gingivitis; for adults it is as much as 90% when all types and causes are included. Gingivitis is very prevalent during pregnancy due to hormonal changes. Other changes in hormonal activity can also increase prevalence of gingivitis in women, including menarche, menstruation, and use of contraceptives.[16]

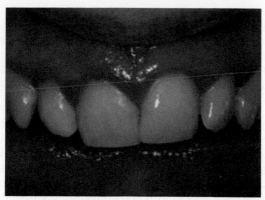

Fig. 2. Gingivitis. (*From* Preshaw PM, Bissett SM. Periodontitis: oral complication of diabetes. Endocrinol Metab Clin North Am 2013;42:849–67; with permission.)

Clinical implications

Gingivitis is often acute but can be intermittent and relapsing; some patients do get chronic gingivitis. Prognosis is generally favorable because it does respond well to appropriate treatment. Some experts think that if left untreated, gingivitis may progress to periodontitis over months to years, which can lead to other issues (see Periodontitis below). There is a condition called acute necrotizing ulcerative gingivitis that includes a necrotic slough of the gingival and is caused by a compromised immune system and malnutrition seen mostly in undeveloped countries.

Box 2
Risk factors for gingivitis

Poor dental hygiene/plaque formation

Eruption of primary or secondary teeth

Dental appliances (dentures, braces)

Malocclusion or dental crowding

Faulty dental restoration

Pregnancy

Uncontrolled diabetes mellitus

Smoking

Mouth breathing

Medications (gingival overgrowth): phenytoin, calcium channel blockers, cyclosporine

Viral illness

HIV-positive, AIDS

Stress; lack of sleep

Hospitalization

Malnutrition

Vitamin C deficiency (scurvy); coenzyme Q10 deficiency

Possible genetic link (up to 30% of population)

Hereditary gingival fibromatosis (rare)

Diagnostic options and dilemmas

Patients report painful gums that bleed easily especially with brushing, flossing, and eating. A thorough history should explore risk factors. Physical examination reveals swollen and erythematous gums that are tender to palpation. Plaque and calculus may be present. Differential includes periodontitis, pericoronitis (a flap of gum tissue growing over a tooth), and other oral ulcerative diseases and infections.

Management

Care should include removing any offending agents (medications, tobacco products) and modify diet if malnutrition is a concern. Dental referrals may be necessary for cleaning and plaque removal or dental appliance refitting. General measures can include warm saline rinses, better oral hygiene, and analgesics if necessary. Chlorhexidine rinses, mouth rinses with essential oils, and fluoridated hydrogen peroxide-based mouth rinses have all been shown to reduce gingivitis significantly.[17,18] Antibiotics are only necessary for acute necrotizing ulcerative gingivitis and include penicillin, metronidazole, and/or erythromycin. Prevention includes good oral hygiene, including daily high-quality flossing[19] and use of an electric toothbrush twice daily,[4] healthy well-rounded diet, and regular dental checkups.

Periodontitis

Description

Periodontitis is a deep inflammation of the gingiva, including the ligaments and supporting structure of the teeth. It is caused by persistent exposure of the mouth to bacteria and plaque, leading to chronic inflammation. (Therefore, like many conditions of the mouth, it is not simply inflammatory but inflammatory and infectious.) Over time this leads to periodontal ligament destruction, loss of supporting alveolar bone, and loosening of teeth. Two major types are chronic and aggressive.

Risk factors

Poor oral hygiene (lack of brushing and flossing) and lack of dental cleanings lead to chronic plaque accumulation. Other contributing factors include tobacco exposure, HIV, pregnancy, and diabetes.[20]

Prevalence

Periodontitis is common. An estimated 20% of adults are affected by periodontitis.[21]

Clinical implications

Periodontitis is the leading cause of tooth loss in adults. Edentulism has been associated with an overall increase in morbidity and mortality.[22] Local infection may also occur resulting in abscess formation. Multiple studies have shown an association between periodontitis and cardiovascular disease, preterm labor, and worsening diabetes among other disease states (although interventions may not improve outcomes making prevention a key goal).[23–25] The inflammation within the mouth leads to a systemic cascade of interleukins and prostaglandins that have wide ranging effects.[26] Interventions to treat periodontitis are not always helpful for the systemic condition (ie, cardiovascular disease, preterm labor) in many studies, raising the question of whether prevention of periodontitis would have a more profound effect.

Diagnostic options and dilemmas

Clinical examination and history reveal painful gums that bleed easily. Advanced disease includes loose teeth. Radiographs show bone loss. Dental assessments to categorize disease will include probing depth of gingiva, attachment loss, and bone loss.

Management

Periodontitis is treated by dental professionals with deep root scaling and planing of bacteria and calculus to address the inflammation deep into the root. Topical antibiotics (metronidazole, minocycline, and doxycycline) and systemic antibiotics (doxycycline 100 mg daily, metronidazole 500 mg twice daily) are also used.[27,28] Chlorhexidine rinses may also be prescribed. Oral hygiene is an essential aspect of management and can be supported by medical professionals. Oral hygiene should include brushing twice daily with fluoridated toothpaste, ideally using an electric oscillating toothbrush, flossing daily, avoiding sugary snacks and drinks, avoiding tobacco products, and regular dental visits and cleanings.

Stomatitis

Description

Stomatitis is an inflammation of the mucous lining of the mouth, which can include the tongue, gingiva, lips, buccal surface, and floor of the mouth. It is usually erythematous and can be ulcerated and usually painful.

Risk factors

Stomatitis can have many causes and therefore there can be many risks, including poor oral hygiene, malnutrition, dietary deficiencies (ie, iron, folic acid, vitamin B6 and B12), chronic systemic disease (ie, inflammatory bowel disease, Behcet disease), immune deficiencies (ie, leukemia, AIDS), poor fitting dentures, smoking, and cancer therapies.[29]

Prevalence

There are no specific estimates of these conditions but the following is a general guideline: very common: herpetic stomatitis (**Fig. 3**), hand-foot-mouth disease, and recurrent aphthous stomatitis; common: herpangina, nicotinic stomatitis, and denture-related stomatitis. The remaining causes are uncommon or rare.

Clinical implications

Most of the common and less serious forms of stomatitis resolve over days to weeks.[30] Resolution is expedited when offending agents are removed (eg, nicotine for nicotinic stomatitis or refitting poorly fitted dentures for denture-related stomatitis).

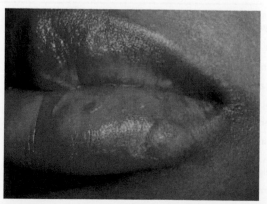

Fig. 3. Herpes simplex stomatitis. (*From* Fatahzadeh M, Schwartz R. Human herpes simplex virus infections: epidemiology, pathogenesis, symptomatology, diagnosis, and management. J Am Acad Dermatol 2007;57(5):737–63; with permission.)

Complications

Complications include intraoral scarring and possible restriction of oral mobility if stomatitis is severe or chronic. Infectious causes can have systemic effects (eg, gangrenous stomatitis leading to facial disfigurement and even death; herpetic stomatitis can be associated with ocular or central nervous system involvement). Systemic disease can also have other systemic effects (eg, Behçet disease may result in vision loss, colitis, vasculitis, large-artery aneurysms, or encephalitis).

Diagnostic options and dilemmas

Patients usually present with complaints of a burning sensation or localized pain (minimal to severe pain), intolerance to temperature changes, and irritation with certain foods. Constitutional symptoms may include low-grade fever, malaise, and headache. Nutrition deficiencies, exposures to medications, foods, or oral products, recent cancer or cancer treatments, nicotine exposure, and systemic symptoms, such as fever, other lesions, or rashes, should be inquired about.

The physical examination should include comprehensive oral examination of all mucosal surfaces. Erythema and edema are the usual oral manifestations. Ulceration can occur in some cases. If *Candida* is involved, a white patch can also be present. Usually no tests are needed. If the diagnosis is in question, the following tests may be helpful: herpes simplex virus culture; serologic testing for syphilis; complete blood count, and cultures to determine secondary infection. A biopsy may be needed for persistent or recurrent lesions. Immunofluorescence is useful in the differential diagnostic between recurrent aphthous stomatitis and bullous skin diseases.

Management

Treatment of stomatitis depends on the cause. If cause is allergic, removal of the agent is critical. For infectious causes, antibiotic or antifungal medications are best. Steroidal anti-inflammatory drugs can help for systemic conditions with stomatitis manifestation. If the cause of stomatitis is due to medical treatment or cancer therapy, therapies may need to be altered.

There are many approaches to providing relief topically in the mouth. See **Box 3**.

Steroids, colchicine, and cytotoxic drugs can be used for Behçet disease. Antibiotics are necessary for gangrenous stomatitis (penicillin and metronidazole are

---

Box 3
Local agents for symptom relief of mouth ulcerations

Acetaminophen or ibuprofen as primary agents for analgesia

2% viscous lidocaine (swish and spit)

Liquid diphenhydramine (swish and spit) for allergic stomatitis

Silver nitrate, 1 application until lesion is white[32]

Topical steroid (Kenalog) in Orabase 3-4 times daily

Dexamethasone ointment 3 times daily[33]

Miracle mouth rinses: various combinations of the following in equal parts (swish and spit) multiple times daily:

    Maalox or Mylanta, diphenhydramine, lidocaine

    Maalox or Mylanta, diphenhydramine, Carafate

    Nystatin, diphenhydramine, hydrocortisone

reasonable first-line agents; often started intravenously). For candidiasis, Nystatin oral suspension (swish and swallow) should be tried. Acyclovir 200 to 800 mg 5 times a day for 7 to 14 days for herpetic stomatitis.

For prevention or reducing severity of mucositis with cancer treatments, these agents have some evidence of benefit: allopurinol, aloe vera, amifostine, cryotherapy, glutamine (intravenous), honey, keratinocyte growth factor, laser, and polymixin/tobramycin/amphotericin antibiotic pastille/paste.[31]

COMMON LESIONS OF THE MOUTH
Bony Tori

Description
Bony tori is a benign bony protuberance that arises from the cortical plate and consists of lamellar bone (**Fig. 4**).[1] They are more common in the hard palate of the mouth but can also occur in the floor of the mouth. They are likely congenital but do not develop until adulthood.

Risk factors
Risk factors include age and possibly family history.

Prevalence
In the United States, the prevalence is approximately 3%, seen slightly more often in women than in men[33] (Palatal tori 25%–35%; mandibular tori 7%–10%).

Clinical implications
Bony tori do not usually cause any symptoms. On occasion, they can cause mechanical interference with eating or denture placement.

Diagnostic options and dilemmas
Tori are usually painless and go unnoticed. Medical personnel can sometimes confuse them for cancerous growths.

Management
No management is necessary unless the tori are interfering with oral function or denture fabrication. An oral surgery consult would be appropriate in these situations.

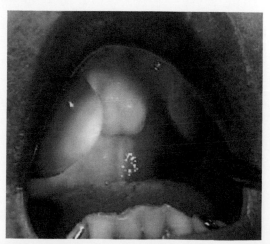

Fig. 4. Bony tori. (*From* Swartz MH. Textbook of physical diagnosis: history and examination. Philadelphia: Saunders; p. 324–61.)

Mucocele

Description
Mucoceles are benign fluid-filled sacs within the lining of the epithelium (**Fig. 5**). They contain mucous glands.

Risk factors
Risk includes mild oral trauma, which leads to disruption of the salivary gland duct.

Prevalence
The prevalence of mucoceles is common and is usually seen in patients under the age of 20.

Clinical implications
The lesions are seldom symptomatic, but often are aggravating because a person will continue to retraumatize them when eating. Patients will present with pinkish/blue soft papules or nodules. Palpation reveals a gelatinous sac usually. Most frequently they occur on the lower lip (ie, result of biting of the lip). They vary in size.

Diagnostic options and dilemmas
Mucoceles are usually easy to diagnose. If there is a lack of gelatinous material, it may simply be gingivitis. Any lesion that does not heal in the mouth over 4 to 6 weeks should be followed up for further assessment and possible biopsy or excision for pathologic evaluation.

Management
Lesions will often rupture spontaneously, which should lead to complete resolution.[34] If the lesions are symptomatic, they can be excised, which must include the entire cyst to prevent recurrence. Aspiration alone is not recommended because it will provide short-term relief but recurrence is common. Alternative treatments include cryosurgery or laser, which also has shown good results with low recurrence rates and the latter being well tolerated.[35]

Lichen Planus

Description
Lichen planus is a chronic inflammatory condition of unknown cause, likely an immune response (**Fig. 6**).

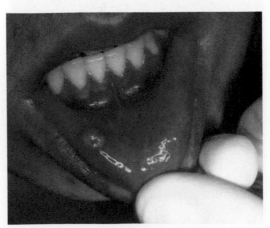

Fig. 5. Mucocele. (*From* Wu CW, Kao YH, Chen CM, et al. Mucoceles of the oral cavity in pediatric patients. Kaohsiung J Med Sci 2011;27(7):276–9; with permission.)

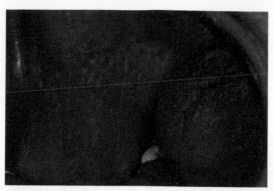

Fig. 6. Lichen planus. (*From* Scully C, Carrozzo M. Oral mucosal disease: Lichen planus. Br J Oral Maxillofac Surg 2008;46:15–21; with permission.)

Risk factors

Ther are no risk factors, possibly age. There may be a genetic link. One proposed theory is that lichen planus is a response to an infection, medication, or trauma.[36]

Prevalence

Lichen planus affects 1% to 2% of the population and can occur at any age but is more predominant over age 40; there is a female-to-male ratio of 1.4:1.[37]

Clinical implications

Clinical implications are benign; however, if not exhibiting classical features or not responding to therapy, they may require a biopsy to confirm diagnosis. Lichen planus occurs at other sites in the body including skin and genitals.

Diagnostic options and dilemmas

Lichen planus are asymptomatic. Usually they will appear like white lace-like striations in the buccal surface. Alternative presentation is an erythematous atropic-appearing lesion; these lesions can be more painful. There is a third type that is more erosive.[38]

Management

Topical medium-to-high potency steroids can be helpful: dry area and apply 3–4 times daily.[39] Goals of management are to decrease pain if present and to prevent scarring. Good oral hygiene, avoiding irritating foods/drinks and tobacco, and removing any appliances that irritate the area may be helpful. Secondary treatments that have some proven benefit include intralesional corticosteroids, cyclosporine, and pimecrolimus and tacrolimus.

Leukoplakia (and Erythroplakia)

Description

Leuokoplakia are premalignant lesions that present as white patches or mucosal thickening (**Fig. 7**). Erythroplakia are similar lesions that have a red or red and white appearance. The lesions are hyperplasia of the squamous epithelium and although they begin as a benign reactive, inflammatory process can also evolve to transformative dysplasia.

Risk factors

The risk factors are similar to oral squamous cell cancers (see Oral Cancer below). Biggest risk factors are carcinogens, especially smokeless tobacco products and

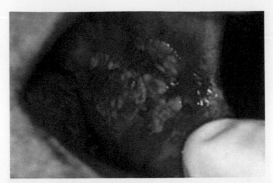

Fig. 7. Leukoplakia and erythroplakia. (*From* Wu CW, Kao YH, Chen CM, et al. Mucoceles of the oral cavity in pediatric patients. Kaohsiung J Med Sci 2011;27(7):276–9; with permission.)

repeat trauma. More evidence is emerging about the role of human papilloma virus (HPV) and leukoplakia.[40]

Prevalence
Benign leukoplakia is common. Erythroplakia is less common. It is estimated that between 1% and 20% of benign lesions become malignant within 10 years.[41]

Clinical implications
White and red lesions in the mouth can be simple trauma, gingivitis, or lichen planus. Areas of the mouth where trauma is common (eg, inside of cheek) have thicker linings and therefore lesions in this area are less likely to be dysplastic. However, traumatic or nontraumatic lesions that do not resolve within 4 weeks should be biopsied. (Note that oral hairy leukoplakia is a different form of mucosal thickening and is not a premalignant lesion. It usually involves the tongue in HIV-infected patients and is not covered in this article.)

Diagnostic options and dilemmas
Usually lesions are asymptomatic and noticed by patients incidentally. (This is the reason periodic examinations by dental and medical professionals can find such lesions before they become more serious.) Lesions will often begin as white or red patches and then progress to thicker plaques or even erosions. Ulcerated lesions are more likely to be cancerous. Clinicians may visualize lesions at any of these stages.

Management
All white or erythematous lesions that cannot be explained or persist should be biopsied.[42] Depending on local expertise, dentists, oral surgeons, and otolaryngologists can perform this procedure. If moderate or severe dysplasia is identified, then surgical excision is the treatment of choice. Mild lesions can be treated with cryotherapy or laser ablation but do not allow for pathologic confirmation of complete removal. Prevention should include advising all patients to avoid tobacco products.

Oral Cancer

Description
Malignancies arising from the lips, tongue, floor of the mouth, salivary glands, buccal mucosa, gums, hard and soft palate, oropharynx, nasopharynx, and hypopharynx or other ill-defined sites within the lip, oral cavity, or pharynx. Ninety percent are

squamous cell carcinomas; the others include lymphomas and adenocarcinomas from minor salivary gland origin and sarcomas.

Risk factors
Seventy-five percent of head and neck cancers are linked to tobacco (smokeless or smoked, including cigars and pipes) and alcohol.[43] Use of both alcohol and tobacco greatly increases risk as compared with those who use tobacco or alcohol alone (synergistic effect). HPV-positive oral cancers has increased by 225% recently and is now responsible for 2.8/100,000 individuals.[44] Ultraviolet light exposures increase risk for cancers of the lips. Radiation exposure from treatment of other facial cancers increases risk of salivary gland cancers. Chronic mechanical irritation (eg, sharp tooth edge, poor-fitting denture) and poor oral hygiene may also contribute. Other possible risk factors include HIV and betal nut chewing (other parts of the world).

Prevalence
Occurrence is 12/100,000/y for oral cancers and when head and neck cancers are taken collectively there are 53,000 new cases annually and 11,500 deaths per year,[45] representing 3% of all cancers in the United States, which is the sixth leading cause of cancer-related mortality. There is 30% to 50% higher incidence in African-Americans than in Caucasians; male > female (2:1); predominant age: >40 years. Oral cancer is the eighth most common cancer worldwide.

Clinical implications
Five-year survival rates have changed very little in the past decade; however, quality of life is much improved.[46] Unfortunately lesions are often detected late. If detected at an early stage, survival from oral cancer is better than 90% at 5 years, whereas late-stage disease survival is only 30%. HPV-related oral cancers have lower recurrence rates than non-HPV-related cancers after excision.

Complications
Complications from disease and treatments include functional and/or cosmetic disabilities proportional to the degree of surgery, location, and stage of tumor. Radiation therapy or chemotherapy can cause stomatitis with or without candidiasis, tissue hypoxia, tongue mucositis, and fibrosis. Xerostomia (dry mouth) is also a common side effect of treatments, which can lead to caries or dysphagia. Radiation may also cause new neoplasms.

Diagnostic options and dilemmas
Clinicians should pay close attention to a history of a nonhealing ulcer or mass in the mouth or on the lip, or any area that bleeds easily or has unexplained pain. Other concerning symptoms may include dysphagia/odynophagia, chronic sore throat or hoarseness, or unexplained ear pain. A thorough oral examination that includes visualization and palpation should be done (and also for those at high risk at regular intervals). Oral cancers can present in many forms. Most concerning are friable granular raised lesions or ulcers that can be confused with infection. Margins may be indurated and hard and extending beyond the borders of the ulcer. A firm neck mass may also suggest metastatic disease. White or red lesions that do not resolve should be biopsied, which is the gold standard for definitive diagnosis. Brush biopsy may be used for smaller oral lesions although, because some studies show brush biopsy to have low sensitivity/specificity, a negative result should be followed with transoral biopsy.[45]

Further imaging is needed for staging. Differential includes stomatitis, infection, benign ulcers, leukoplakia, and lichen planus.

Management

Treatment varies depending on the location. Surgery and radiotherapy for early disease are comparable. Primary radiotherapy (and/or chemotherapy for palliation) is suggested for unresectable tumors and patients not amenable to surgery.

A dental consult should be obtained before any treatment to prevent serious complications later and to treat or eliminate questionable tooth and gum disease. The severity of mucositis during treatment can be lessened with aloe vera, amifostine, cryotherapy, granulocyte colony stimulating factor, intravenous glutamine, honey, keratinocyte growth factor, laser, polymyxin/tobramycin/amphotericin, antibiotic pastille/paste, and sucralfate.[47] Avoidance of risk factors for secondary prevention and periodic surveillance examinations are important.[48]

SUMMARY

There are a host of diseases that manifest in the mouth primarily or secondarily. Medical clinicians should become familiar with presentations for common and serious conditions as outlined above. Clinicians can often make initial diagnosis and management decisions and then refer as necessary. Often a team approach is needed for more complex or chronic conditions. Primary care providers can play an important role in prevention and early diagnosis by advising patients to perform proper hygiene and avoid tobacco and excess alcohol, have regular dental checkups, minimize prescribing medications with oral effects, promote a healthy diet, examine the oral cavity periodically, and make timely referrals.

REFERENCES

1. Bouquot JE. Bond's book of oral disease. 4th edition. The Maxillofacial Center for Diagnostic and Research; 2001. Available at: http://www.maxillofacialcenter.com/BondBook/bone/exostosis.html. Accessed February 20, 2013.
2. Selwitz RH, Ismail AI, Pitts NB. Dental caries. Lancet 2007;369(9555):51.
3. Dye BA, Li X, Beltrán-Aguilar ED. Selected oral health indicators in the United States, 2005–2008. NCHS data brief, no 96. Hyattsville (MD): National Center for Health Statistics; 2012.
4. Marinho VC. Topical fluoride (toothpastes, mouthrinses, gels or varnishes) for preventing dental caries in children and adolescents. Cochrane Oral Health Group. Cochrane Database Syst Rev 2007;(4):CD002781.
5. Robinson PG, Deacon SA, Deery C, et al. Manual versus powered toothbrushing for oral health. Cochrane Database Syst Rev 2005;(2):CD002281. http://dx.doi.org/10.1002/14651858.CD002281.pub2.
6. Douglass AB, Douglass JM. Common dental emergencies. Am Fam Physician 2003;67:511–6.
7. Matijevic S, Lazi Z, Kuljic-Kapulica N, et al. Empirical antimicrobial therapy of acute dentoalveolar abscess. Vojnosanit Pregl 2009;66:544–50.
8. Hurley MC, Heran MK. Imaging studies for head and neck infections. Infect Dis Clin North Am 2007;21(2):305.
9. Cliff K. An evidence-based update of the use of analgesics in dentistry. Periodontol 2000 2008;46(1):143–64.
10. Akpan A, Morgan R. Oral candidiasis. Postgrad Med J 2002;78:455–9.
11. Yang IA, Clarke MS, Sim EH, et al. Inhaled corticosteroids for stable chronic obstructive pulmonary disease. Cochrane Database Syst Rev 2012;(7):CD002991.
12. Oral candidiasis statistics. Centers for Disease Control and Prevention. National Center for Emerging and Zoonotic Infectious Diseases, Division of Foodborne,

Waterborne, and Environmental Diseases. Available at: www.cdc.gov/fungal/candidiasis/thrush/statistics.html. Accessed February 20, 2013.

13. Pappas PG, Kauffman CA, Andes D, et al. Clinical practice guidelines for the management of candidiasis: 2009 update by the Infectious Diseases Society of America. Clin Infect Dis 2009;48:503–35.

14. Kanli A, Demirel F, Sezgin Y. Oral candidosis, denture cleanliness and hygiene habits in an elderly population. Aging Clin Exp Res 2005;17(6):502.

15. Armitage GC. Development of a classification system for periodontal diseases and conditions. Ann Periodontol 1999;4(1):1.

16. Mariotti A. Dental plaque-induced gingival diseases. Ann Periodontol 1999;4(1):7.

17. Stoeken JE, Paraskevas S, van der Weijden GA. The long-term effect of a mouthrinse containing essential oils on dental plaque and gingivitis: a systematic review. J Periodontol 2007;78(7):1218–28.

18. Gunsolley JC. Clinical efficacy of antimicrobial mouthrinses. J Dent 2010; 38(Suppl 1):S6–10.

19. Sambunjak D, Nickerson JW, Poklepovic T, et al. Flossing for the management of periodontal diseases and dental caries in adults. Cochrane Database Syst Rev 2011;(12):CD008829.

20. Taylor GW. Bidirectional interrelationships between diabetes and periodontal diseases: an epidemiologic perspective. Ann Periodontol 2001;6(1):99.

21. Eke PI, Dye BA, Wei L, et al. Prevalence of periodontitis in adults in the United States: 2009 and 2010. CDC Periodontal Disease Surveillance workgroup. J Dent Res 2012;91(10):914.

22. Brown DW. Complete edentulism prior to the age of 65 years is associated with all-cause mortality. J Public Health Dent 2009;69(4):260–6.

23. Friedewald VE, Kornman KS, Beck JD, et al. The American Journal of Cardiology and J Periodontol editors' consensus: periodontitis and atherosclerotic cardiovascular disease. J Periodontol 2009;80(7):1021–32.

24. Southerland JH, Taylor GW, Moss K, et al. Commonality in chronic inflammatory diseases: periodontitis, diabetes, and coronary artery disease. Periodontol 2000 2006;40(1):130–43.

25. Xiong X, Buekens P, Fraser WD, et al. Periodontal disease and adverse pregnancy outcomes: a systematic review. BJOG 2006;113(2):135–43.

26. Kumar J, Samelson R. Oral health care during pregnancy and early childhood practice guidelines. New York: New York State Department of Health; 2006.

27. Eberhard J, Jepsen S, Jervøe-Storm PM, et al. Full-mouth disinfection for the treatment of adult chronic periodontitis. Cochrane Database Syst Rev 2008;(1):CD004622. http://dx.doi.org/10.1002/14651858.CD004622.pub2.

28. Krayer JW, Leite RS, Kirkwood KL. Non-surgical chemotherapeutic treatment strategies for the management of periodontal diseases. Dent Clin North Am 2010;54(1):13.

29. McBride DR. Management of aphthous ulcers. Am Fam Physician 2000;62(1):149.

30. Ship JA. Recurrent aphthous stomatitis. An update. Oral Surg Oral Med Oral Pathol Oral Radiol Endod 1996;81(2):141.

31. Worthington HV, Clarkson JE, Bryan G, et al. Interventions for preventing oral mucositis for patients with cancer receiving treatment. Cochrane Database Syst Rev 2010;(12):CD000978.

32. Alidaee MR, Taheri A, Mansoori P, et al. Silver nitrate cautery in aphthous stomatitis: a randomized controlled trial. Br J Dermatol 2005;153(3):521.

33. Liu C, Zhou Z, Liu G, et al. Efficacy and safety of dexamethasone ointment on recurrent aphthous ulceration. Am J Med 2012;125(3):292–301.

34. Chi AC, Lambert PR III, Richardson MS, et al. Oral mucoceles: a clinicopathologic review of 1,824 cases, including unusual variants. J Oral Maxillofac Surg 2011;69(4):1086–93.
35. Huang IY, Chen CM, Kao YH, et al. Treatment of mucocele of the lower lip with carbon dioxide laser. J Oral Maxillofac Surg 2007;65(5):855.
36. Roopashree MR, Gondhalekar RV, Shashikanth MC, et al. Pathogenesis of oral lichen planus–a review. J Oral Pathol Med 2010;39(10):729–34.
37. McCartan BE, Healy CM. The reported prevalence of oral lichen planus: a review and critique. J Oral Pathol Med 2008;37(8):447–53.
38. Eisen D. The clinical manifestations and treatment of oral lichen planus. Dermatol Clin 2003;21(1):79–89.
39. Thongprasom K, Carrozzo M, Furness S, et al. Interventions for treating oral lichen planus. Cochrane Database Syst Rev 2011;(7):CD001168. http://dx.doi.org/10.1002/14651858.CD001168.pub2.
40. Cianfriglia F, Di Gregorio DA, Cianfriglia C, et al. Incidence of human papillomavirus infection in oral leukoplakia. Indications for a viral aetiology. J Exp Clin Cancer Res 2006;25(1):21.
41. Lee JJ, Hong WK, Hittelman WN, et al. Predicting cancer development in oral leukoplakia: ten years of translational research. Clin Cancer Res 2000;6(5):1702.
42. van der Waal I, Schepman KP, van der Meij EH. A modified classification and staging system for oral leukoplakia. Oral Oncol 2000;36(3):264.
43. Blot WJ, McLaughlin JK, Winn DM, et al. Smoking and drinking in relation to oral and pharyngeal cancer. Cancer Res 1988;48(11):3282.
44. Chaturvedi AK, Engels RA, Pfeiffer RM, et al. Human papilloma virus and rising incidence of oropharangeal cancer incidence in the United States. J Clin Oncol 2011;29(32):4294–301.
45. Siegel R, Naishadham D, Jemal A. Cancer statistics, 2013. CA Cancer J Clin 2013;63(1):11–30.
46. Genden EM, Ferlito A, Silver CL, et al. Contemroary management of cancer of the oral cavity. Eur Arch Otorhinolaryngol 2010;267:1001–17.
47. Worthington HV, Clarkson JE, Bryan G, et al. Interventions for preventing oral mucositis for patients with cancer receiving treatment. Cochrane Database Syst Rev 2011;(4):CD000978.
48. Brocklehurst P, Kujan O, Glenny AM, et al. Screening programmes for the early detection and prevention of oral cancer. Cochrane Database Syst Rev 2010;(11):CD004150.

Pharyngitis

Ruth Weber, MD, MSEd

KEYWORDS

- Pharyngitis • Throat • Infectious • Noninfectious

KEY POINTS

- Most infectious pharyngitis has a viral cause, which includes influenza, coronavirus, rhinovirus, adenovirus, enterovirus, human immunodeficiency virus, Epstein-Barr virus, cytomegalovirus, and herpes simplex virus.
- The clinician must quickly rule out parapharyngeal space infections, peritonsilar abscess, submandibular abscess (Ludwig angina), and epiglottitis. These conditions require emergency care.
- The Infectious Diseases Society of America advises the use of aspirin or nonsteroidal anti-inflammatory agents (NSAIAs) in adults and NSAIAs in children for the treatment of pain. There are several studies that show that NSAIAs relieve pharyngitis pain better than acetaminophen.
- Penicillin remains the antibiotic of choice of group A beta-hemolytic streptococcal (GAS) pharyngitis. Resistance has not developed to penicillin.
- Patients with GAS pharyngitis should have improvement in 3 to 4 days. If not better at that time, the patient should be seen for diagnostic reconsideration or the development of a suppurative complication.

INTRODUCTION

Sore throat is common and has substantial medical and societal costs. There were more than 15 million outpatient visits for pharyngitis in 2007 in the United States.[1] Overtreatment of non–group A beta-hemolytic streptococcal (GAS) infections is one of the major causes of inappropriate use of antibiotics. Patient's expectations are not for antibiotics, but for pain relief, reassurance, and information. When questioned, those who hoped for an antibiotic did so with the belief that an antibiotic would give pain relief. Therefore, it behooves the medical provider to have a rational, practical, and evidence-based approach to the treatment of pharyngitis.

CAUSES/EPIDEMIOLOGY OF PHARYNGITIS

The causes of pharyngitis may be categorized as infectious versus noninfectious. Infectious causes are shown in **Table 1**. Noninfectious causes include allergy, postnasal

Department of Family and Community Medicine, University of Kansas School of Medicine-Wichita, 1010 North Kansas, Wichita, KS 67214, USA
E-mail address: ruth.weber@wesleymc.com

Prim Care Clin Office Pract 41 (2014) 91–98
http://dx.doi.org/10.1016/j.pop.2013.10.010
0095-4543/14/$ – see front matter © 2014 Elsevier Inc. All rights reserved.

Table 1
Infectious causes of pharyngitis

Bacteria	Viruses	Atypical Bacteria
Group A beta-hemolytic streptococci	Adenovirus	*Mycoplasma pneumoniae*
Group C streptococci	Herpes simplex virus 1 and 2	*Chlamydophila pneumoniae*
Neisseria gonorrhoeae	Coxsackievirus	*Chlamydophila psittaci*
Corynebacterium diphtheriae	Rhinovirus	—
Fusobacterium necrophorum	Coronavirus	—
Francisella tularensis	Influenza A and B	—
Yersinia pestis	Parainfluenza	—
Treponema pallidum	Respiratory syncytial virus	—
Mixed anaerobes	Human herpes virus 4 (Epstein-Barr virus)	—
—	Human herpes virus 5 (Cytomegalovirus)	—
—	HIV	—

Abbreviation: HIV, human immunodeficiency virus.
Data from Kociolek L, Shulman S. Pharyngitis. Ann Intern Med 2013;157(5):ITC3-1.

drainage, irritation (ie, smoke exposure, poorly humidified air), gastrointestinal reflux disease, foreign body, acute thyroiditis, and referred pain (ie, dental).[2] Infectious causes include viral and bacterial.[2] In the immune-compromised patient, fungal causes should be considered.[2] The most important of these infections is GAS because of the possible complications.

Most infectious pharyngitis has a viral cause, which includes influenza, coronavirus, rhinovirus, adenovirus, enterovirus, human immunodeficiency virus (HIV), Epstein-Barr virus (EBV), cytomegalovirus, and herpes simplex virus.[2]

The major risk factors for GAS are age and exposure. Up to 30% of childhood pharyngitis is caused by GAS. Outbreaks occur during winter and early spring in the 5-year-old to 15-year-old age group, and spread by close contact (school and home). GAS is uncommon in preschool-aged children and adults. Group C and G beta-hemolytic *Streptococcus* causes pharyngitis in older children and adults.[3] The infection is similar but less severe and does not lead to the significant complications of GAS infection. Consider mycoplasma and chlamydia infections when young adults present with pharyngitis and bronchitis.[4]

Fusobacterium necrophorum (Fn), an obligate anaerobic gram-negative bacillus, has been reported as causing pharyngitis in adolescents in the United Kingdom and Denmark.[3] Although not a conclusive pathogen for pharyngitis, it has been suggested as a causative agent in Lemierre syndrome (septic thrombophlebitis of the internal jugular vein with septic emboli to the lungs).

HISTORY AND PHYSICAL EXAMINATION

The physical examination of the patient is focused on the head/neck/chest and skin. On initial examination, the provider should assess for signs of life-threatening disease, especially in children who have difficulty in localizing pain. Red flags for impending life-threatening deterioration include difficulty with handling secretions, drooling, hot-potato voice, toxic appearance, and unilateral neck swelling.[1] The clinician must quickly rule out parapharyngeal space infections, peritonsilar abscess, submandibular abscess (Ludwig angina), and epiglottitis. These conditions require emergency care.[1]

Viral Pharyngitis

Patients complain of sore throat, nasal congestion, coryza, hoarseness, sinus discomfort, ear pain, cough, conjunctivitis, diarrhea, and discrete ulcerative stomatitis. Herpangina (Coxsackie virus) manifests with fever and painful vesicular lesions in the posterior oropharynx. Hand, foot, and mouth disease (Coxsackie A-16) has painful vesicles and ulcers in the mouth, palms, and soles.

Infectious Mononucleosis

Patients present with a classic triad of severe sore throat, diffuse lymphadenopathy, and fever (up to 40°C [104°F]). Up to 90% of cases are caused by infection with human herpesvirus 4, more commonly known as EBV. The remaining 10% of cases are caused by cytomegalovirus (herpes virus 5) and herpes virus 6. There is a prodrome of chills, sweats, fever, and malaise. One-third of patients present with exudates and palatal petechiae that may mimic GAS infection. Approximately 15% of patients present with jaundice and 5% with a rash. Up to one-third of adults and adolescents have significant illness, whereas most children have subclinical infection. Patients with mononucleosis who ingest a β-lactam antibiotic often develop a pruritic maculopapular rash.

Acute Retroviral Syndrome

Primary HIV infection can mimic EBV infection. Patients present with fever, nonexudative pharyngitis, weight loss, and diffuse adenopathy. Between 40% and 80% of patients develop a rash 2 weeks after infection.

GAS Pharyngitis

GAS pharyngitis classically presents with sudden onset of severe sore throat, pain on swallowing, and fever without cough or rhinorrhea. Clinical signs include tonsillar erythema with or without exudate, anterior cervical adenitis, soft palate petechiae, red swollen uvula, and scarlatiniform rash. Patents with GAS may have milder symptoms and clinical signs after tonsillectomy.

Streptococcosis

Children less than 3 years of age with group B streptococcal infection may present with atypical symptoms. They have low-grade fever, tender anterior adenopathy, and nasal congestion/discharge. Nonsuppurative complications are rare and the only benefit to treating these children is to decrease transmission. The Infectious Diseases Society of America (IDSA) and the American Pediatric Academy (APA) do not recommend testing these children unless other risk factors are present.[5]

Scarlet Fever

Scarlet fever is GAS pharyngitis infection with a bacterial strain that produces erythrogenic toxins. There is a characteristic fine, goose-pimple red rash that blanches with pressure. The rash begins on the neck and spreads to the trunk and extremities, sparing the face. It is more pronounced in creases. The rash fades in 3 to 4 days and the skin may have subsequent desquamation.

DIAGNOSIS

Expert clinicians cannot reliably identify patients infected with GAS, therefore microbiologic confirmation is necessary to diagnose GAS pharyngitis. Several prediction tools for determining the probability of GAS infection have been proposed. The IDSA recommends the use of a clinical scoring system to reduce unnecessary testing and treatment.[5] The Centor Criteria (for adults) was modified by McIssac and colleagues[6] to include an age criterion, and has expanded the applicability of the tool to all ages (**Table 2**).[7]

Those with 0 to 1 criterion are considered low risk and do not require additional evaluation or antibiotic treatment.[7] Those with 2 to 3 criteria should be assessed for GAS and treated only if positive.[7] Guidelines for management of patients with 4 criteria differ. Although the American College of Physicians (ACP) recommends empiric treatment of individuals with 4 positive criteria, the IDSA and the American Heart Association (AHA) do not.[5] Routine empiric treatment of GAS in patients with 4 criteria increases unnecessary use of antibiotics by up to 50%.[7]

If the clinical symptoms suggest GAS infection, throat culture, rapid antigen detection testing (RADT), or DNA probe testing is indicated.[8–10] The specimen should be obtained before the initiation of antibiotics, because even 1 dose can cause the test to be negative. Both tonsils and the posterior pharynx should be aggressively swabbed. Other areas of the mouth should be avoided with the swab.

In children, a throat culture should be performed if the RADT is negative in order to identify patients who have a false-negative result. In adults, the throat culture is not necessary after a negative RADT because of the low incidence of GAS and low risk of acute rheumatic fever (RF).[8] Some laboratories are replacing throat culture conformation with DNA probe testing. The turnaround time is 24 hours, compared with 48 hours with throat culture. There is no value in obtaining streptococcal antibody testing (antistreptolysin O [ASO]) and antideoxyribonuclease B during acute GAS infection. This testing is only needed to diagnose acute RF.

Acute Mononucleosis

With acute mononucleosis, a complete blood count shows an absolute lymphocytosis with greater than 10% atypical lymphocytes. Within 2 to 3 weeks the heterophile antibody test becomes positive. Because of a higher false-negative rate in children, an EBV-specific antibody may be necessary for diagnosis.

Acute Retroviral Syndrome

A presumptive diagnosis of acute retroviral syndrome is made with HIV antigen detection (HIV antibodies may be negative). An HIV viral load assay of more than 10,000 copies/mL confirms the diagnosis.

Table 2 Modified centor criteria	
Fever	1 point
Absence of cough	1 point
Anterior cervical adenitis	1 point
Tonsillar exudate	1 point
Age (y)	
2–14	1 point
15–44	0 point
45 or older	−1 point

Group C and G Streptococci

Consider group C and G streptococcal infection when an RADT/culture is negative and the patient continues to have severe symptoms. Diagnosis requires throat culture with special notice to the laboratory of specific strains of interest because many laboratories ignore them in culture.

Fn

Fn is confirmed by growth of Fn bacteria in an anaerobic blood culture.

Treatment

Symptom relief, especially of pain, is the goal of treatment. Patients with confirmed GAS infection should be given antibiotics.

Topical treatment

Salt-water gargles, phenol throat sprays, and herbal remedies are often recommended, but there are no studies to recommend or discourage the practice. Sipping warm or cold beverages has been advocated, but honey should be avoided in those less than I year of age because of the concern regarding botulism. Both ambroxol and lidocaine lozenges are significantly better than placebo in providing pain relief without adverse effects.[11] Benzocaine lozenges also provide pain relief; however, the US Food and Drug Administration has published concerns about the risk of methemoglobinemia with their use.[11] Oral rinse with equal parts lidocaine, diphenhydramine, and Maalox may be helpful in patients with stomatitis, gingivitis, and ulcers.[11] It is important for the patient to swish and expectorate to avoid overdose of lidociane.[11]

Systemic analgesics

The IDSA advises the use of aspirin or nonsteroidal antiinflammatory agents (NSAIA) in adults and NSAIAs in children for the treatment of pain.[5] There are several studies that show that NSAIA relieve pharyngitis pain better than acetaminophen.

The use of glucocorticoids for the treatment of pharyngitis is controversial. The IDSA recommends against the use of glucocorticoids for decreasing the duration of pain.[5] Glucocorticoids should be restricted to the exceptional patient with severe sore throat or inability to swallow.[12,13] A single dose of oral dexamethasone of 0.6 mg/kg, maximum of 10 mg is recommended.[14] In adults, a single dose of prednisone 60 mg for 1 to 2 days is acceptable.[12]

Antibiotics

GAS Penicillin remains the antibiotic of choice of GAS pharyngitis (**Table 3**). Resistance has not developed to penicillin. There are strains of GAS that have developed tolerance with minimal inhibitory concentration greater than 32. The clinical significance of this is unknown. Amoxicillin can replace penicillin for treatment, because it has a better taste than penicillin in the oral form. In patients allergic to penicillin, a first-generation cephalosporin or macrolide may be substituted. There are high rates of resistance to macrolides. Antibiotics should be given for 10 days to eradicate GAS from the pharynx.[15] At this time, short-course treatment cannot be recommended except for cefpodoxime, cefdinir, or azithromycin.[15]

In most European guidelines, treatment of GAS is with symptomatic treatment alone.[16] It is considered a self-limiting disease and antibiotics are not commonly recommended because they provide only moderate clinical benefits in a disease with low complication rates. Antibiotics are only prescribed for severe cases. There is a growing body of evidence that treating all patients with GAS pharyngitis to prevent a rare case of RF is not clinically prudent.[8] Penicillin anaphylaxis occurs in approximately

Table 3
Treatment regimens for GAS pharyngitis

Medication	Dosage	Frequency	Duration
Penicillin VK	40 mg/kg/d up to adult dose of 1000 mg/d	Two to 3 times a day	10 d
Amoxicillin	50 mg/kg/d up to adult dose of 1000 mg/d	Twice daily	10 d
Moxatag	750 mg/d (more than 12 y of age)	Daily	10 d
Penicillin G Benzathine	Weight <27 kg, 600,000 units Weight >27 kg, 1.2 million units	Intramuscular once	—
Use for patients who are unlikely to complete a full course of oral medications and for those with a personal or family history of RF			
First-generation cephalosporin	25–50 mg/kg/d up to adult dose of 1000 mg/d	Twice daily	10 d
Erythromycin	20–40 mg/kg/d up to adult dose of 1000 mg/d	Three to 4 times daily	10 d
Azithromycin	Day 1: 10 mg/kg up to adult dose of 500 mg Days 2–5: 5 mg/kg up to adult dose of 250 mg/d	Daily	Days
Dosage is not established for infants younger than 6 mo.			

0.015% of patients, with a fatality rate from shock of 0.002%. Overall morbidity from 10 days of antibiotics may be as high as 10%.

Group C or G beta-hemolytic *Streptococcus* Use the same doses as for GAS but treat for 5 days.

Fn Treatment of pharyngitis is controversial. Some clinicians recommend consideration of treating patients between 15 and 30 years of age with 3 or more Centor Criteria with penicillin or a cephalosporin. It is uncertain whether this treatment is effective for prevention of Lemierre syndrome.

FOLLOW-UP

Patients with GAS pharyngitis should have improvement in 3 to 4 days. If not better at that time, the patient should be seen for diagnostic reconsideration or the development of a suppurative complication.

A test of cure (either RADT or throat culture) is only indicated if the patient has a personal history of RF, develops GAS during RF or after streptococcal glomerulonephritis outbreak, or there is recurrent spread among family members.[17]

RECURRENT GAS PHARYNGITIS

Patients who have repeated symptomatic episodes of GAS are either carriers of GAS with recurrent viral infections, have nonadherence to antibiotic therapy, have new GAS infection, or are (rarely) a treatment failure. When a patient experiences a second episode of GAS after a short interval, the practitioner should repeat the course of therapy with an antibiotic with greater β-lactamase stability or treat with intramuscular penicillin. It is not recommended to obtain RADT or throat culture after the second course of antibiotics. If there is a concern that GAS is being spread among close contacts, all close contacts should be tested for GAS and those who are positive should be treated. Family pets are not reservoirs and do not spread GAS.

The IDSA does not recommend tonsillectomy solely to reduce the frequency of GAS pharyngitis.[5] Tonsillectomy provides a short-lived benefit for a small fraction of patients.[18] However, many clinicians consider tonsillectomy if a child is severely affected by GAS pharyngitis (ie, 7 or more documented GAS infections within 1 year, 5 or more within 2 years, or 3 or more within 3 years).[18] Other indications for tonsillectomy include tonsillar obstruction, recurrent peritonsillar abscess, and chronic GAS carrier in close contact with a patient who has had RF.[18]

GAS Carrier

Up to 20% of children are GAS carriers. The clinician should suspect a GAS carrier when the clinical picture is of viral pharyngitis but patients have positive RADT or throat culture when both symptomatic and asymptomatic. They have no serologic response to ASO and anti-DNase B and have very low risk for complications. They do not need to be identified or treated. There is no need to attempt to eradicate GAS from the pharynx and they do not spread disease to others.

COMPLICATIONS

Complications from GAS pharyngitis are classified as suppurative and nonsuppurative. Nonsuppurative complications include acute RF, acute poststreptococcal glomerulonephritis (poststrep GN) and poststreptococcal reactive arthritis. RF is rare in developed countries. In the United States, the last RF epidemic was in 1985. It occurs 2 to 3 weeks after GAS pharyngitis and is not seen after skin infection. RF is diagnosed using the Revised Jones Criteria for acute RF. Starting antibiotics within 9 days of symptoms can prevent acute RF. Acute poststrep GN occurs approximately 10 days after pharyngeal infection and up to 21 days after skin infection. Antibiotics do not alter the attack rate. Poststreptococcal reactive arthritis is similar to other reactive arthritis and is not altered by antibiotics.

Suppurative complications include peritonsillar abscess, retropharyngeal abscess, sinusitis, otitis media, and mastoiditis. Appropriate treatment of GAS pharyngitis may decrease these complications.

Pediatric Autoimmune Neuropsychiatric Disorder Associated with Group A Streptococci

Pediatric autoimmune neuropsychiatric disorder associated with Group A streptococci (PANDAS) is a controversial diagnosis of children whose obsessive-compulsive disorder or tic disorder is worsened by GAS infection.

REFERENCES

1. Wessels MR. Streptococcal pharyngitis. N Engl J Med 2011;264(7):648–55.
2. Kociolek L, Shulman S. Pharyngitis. Ann Intern Med 2013;157(5):ITC3-1.
3. Centor R. Adolescent and adult pharyngitis: more than "strep throat": comment on "large-scale validation of the Centor and McIsaac scores to predict group A streptococcal pharyngitis". Available at: http://archinte.jamanetwork.com/article.aspx?articleid=1157414. Accessed October 7, 2012.
4. Mitchell M, Sorrentino A, Centor R. Adolescent pharyngitis: a review of bacterial causes. Clin Pediatr 2011;50:1091. Available at: http://cpj.sagepub.com/content/50/12/1091.

5. Shulman S, Bisno A, Clegg HW, et al. Clinical practice guideline for the diagnosis and management of group a streptococcal pharyngitis: 2012 update by the Infectious Diseases Society of America. Clin Infect Dis 2012;55(10):e86–102.
6. McIsaac WJ, White D, Tannenbaum D, et al. A clinical score to reduce unnecessary antibiotic use in patients with sore throat. CMAJ 1998;15(1):75–83.
7. McIsaac W, Dellner J, Aufricht P, et al. Empirical validation of guidelines for the management of pharyngitis in children and adults. JAMA 2004;291(13):1587–94.
8. Pelucchi C, Grigoryan L, Galeone C, et al, ESCMID Sore Throat Guideline Group. Guideline for the management of acute sore throat. Clin Microbiol Infect 2012; 18(Suppl 1):1–28. Available at: http://www.ncbi.nlm.nih.gov/pubmed/22432746.
9. Matthys J, De Meyere M, van Driel ML, et al. Differences among international pharyngitis guidelines: not just academic. Ann Fam Med 2007;5(5):436–46. Available at: www.annfammed.org.
10. Frye R, Bailey J, Blevins A. Which treatments provide the most relief for pharyngitis pain? J Fam Pract 2011;60(5):293–4.
11. McNally D, Shephard A, Field E. Randomised, double-blind, placebo-controlled study of a single dose of amylmetacrestol/2,4-dichlorobenzl alcohol plus lidocaine lozenge or a hexylresorcinol lozenge for the treatment of acute sore throat due to upper respiratory tract infection. J Pharm Pharm Sci 2012;15(2):281–94.
12. Hayward G, Thompson MJ, Perera R, et al. Corticosteroids as standalone or add-on treatment from sore throat [review]. Cochrane Database Syst Rev 2012;(10):CD008268.
13. American Academy of Pediatrics Committee on Infectious Disease. Red book. 28th edition. Elk Grove Village (IL): American Academy of Pediatrics; 2009.
14. Schams SC, Goldman RD. Steroids as adjuvant treatment of sore throat in acute bacterial pharyngitis. Can Fam Physician 2012;58(1):52–4.
15. Altamini S, Khalil A, Khalaiwi KA, et al. Short-term late-generation antibiotics versus longer term penicillin for acute streptococcal pharyngitis in children. Cochrane Database Syst Rev 2012;(8):CD004872.
16. Chiappini E, Principi N, Mansi N, et al. Management of acute pharyngitis in children: summary of the Italian National Institute of Health Guidelines. Clin Ther 2012;34(6):1442–58.e2.
17. Nakhoul G, Hickner J. Management of adults with acute streptococcal pharyngitis: minimal value for backup strep testing and overuse of antibiotics. J Gen Intern Med 2013;28(6):830–4.
18. Isaacson G. Tonsillectomy care for the pediatrician. Pediatrics 2012;120(2):324–34.

Laryngeal Problems

Scott E. Moser, MD

KEYWORDS

- Laryngopharyngeal reflux • Larynx • Endoscopy • Hoarseness • Vocal cord

KEY POINTS

- Chronic hoarseness is the most common presenting concern for patients with laryngeal pathologic abnormality.
- Chronic hoarseness lasting longer than 3 weeks merits visualization of the vocal cords, especially in smokers because of the potential for carcinoma.
- Early diagnosis and treatment are important for improving outcomes in patients with laryngeal carcinoma.
- As many as half of patients with laryngeal and voice disorders have laryngopharyngeal reflux (LPR).
- Most patients with LPR do not have classic gastroesophageal reflux disease symptoms, so treatment must be more aggressive and prolonged.
- Visualization of the hypopharynx and larynx is best accomplished via flexible nasolaryngoscopy.

INTRODUCTION

Laryngeal complaints are common reasons for patients to seek care in family medicine offices. There is considerable overlap between patient symptoms, such as hoarseness and chronic cough, and final diagnosis, such as laryngopharyngeal reflux (LPR) or laryngeal carcinoma. Therefore, this article begins with a general approach to laryngeal symptoms followed by individual consideration of both the common and serious conditions of the larynx. The focus is on adults because children who present with chronic laryngeal complaints are usually younger than 3 years of age, too young to cooperate with office evaluation, thus requiring initial specialist referral.[1]

Elderly patients have a high prevalence of voice problems but often assume they are a natural part of aging. However, the voice problem can negatively affect quality of life and socialization, particularly when combined with hearing problems. Many voice problems are treatable; therefore, physicians can meaningfully intervene when, in the course of comprehensive care of elderly patients, they recognize and offer treatment options to elderly patients with voice findings.[2]

Department of Family and Community Medicine, University of Kansas School of Medicine–Wichita, 1010 North Kansas, Wichita, KS 67214, USA
E-mail address: smoser@kumc.edu

Prim Care Clin Office Pract 41 (2014) 99–107
http://dx.doi.org/10.1016/j.pop.2013.10.008
0095-4543/14/$ – see front matter © 2014 Elsevier Inc. All rights reserved.

PATIENT HISTORY

Patients with a laryngeal pathologic condition present most commonly with chronic hoarseness. This may be the classic raspy, weak voice or may be more subtle dysphonia as in easy voice fatigue or loss of singing range. Acute hoarseness is a common symptom of self-limited upper respiratory infections. Chronic hoarseness typically means longer than 3 weeks, the usual time by which the symptoms from acute respiratory infections should have resolved. After 3 weeks, the likelihood of a significant pathologic condition increases and thorough evaluation is indicated. This is especially true in smokers because of the increased incidence of laryngeal cancer and the importance of early definitive treatment to achieve a good outcome.[3]

Other common presenting symptoms include chronic cough, globus or foreign-body sensation, chronic sore throat, and frequent throat clearing. People in occupations that depend on the use of their voice are most likely to present for voice concerns and are often the patients at greatest risk of vocal abuse, including teachers, public speakers, singers, and so forth.

PHYSICAL EXAMINATION

The hypopharynx and larynx cannot be visualized on standard physical examination, so special instruments are required. Classically, the examiner used a combination of a lamp behind the patient aligned with a head mirror aligned with a right-angle laryngeal mirror inserted past the patient's tongue to gain an indirect view. Now the examination can be accomplished directly via flexible nasolaryngoscopy.

In addition to visualization of the hypopharynx and larynx, physical examination should include a thorough head and neck examination focusing on potential signs of chronic inflammation or irritation, such as sinusitis or allergic rhinitis, and potential neoplasia, such as masses under the tongue or on the thyroid or cervical lymph nodes.

ANATOMY

To address laryngeal problems, first it is important to understand the anatomy. **Fig. 1** outlines the key anatomic structures of the larynx. The figure is oriented with anterior at the bottom, the way the larynx appears through the nasolaryngoscope instead of the traditional anterior at the top orientation of anatomy texts and imaging studies. Key anterior landmarks include the vallecula and epiglottis. The primary landmarks posteriorly are the

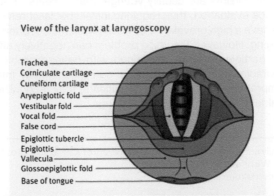

Fig. 1. Laryngeal anatomy. (*Modified from* Burdett E, Mitchell V. Anatomy of the larynx, trachea, and bronchi. Anesthesia & Intensive Care Medicine 2008;9(8):329–33; with permission.)

paired arytenoid cartilages; the corniculate cartilages are the most posterior and medial, and the cuneiforms are slightly anterior and lateral. These serve as attachment sites for the laryngeal muscles involved in the complex control of the vocal cords required for phonation. Innervation of these muscles is primarily from the recurrent laryngeal nerves, so any lesion along their course from the upper chest can cause hoarseness.

The true vocal cords are thin bands of muscle and fibrous tissue covered by squamous epithelium, stretching between the thyroid cartilage anteriorly and the arytenoids posteriorly to form a symmetric "V" with the base anterior. Asymmetry is pathologic. Just lateral to the true vocal cords are the false cords, covered by columnar epithelium. The canal running between the true vocal cords and false cords forms an epithelial transition zone termed the laryngeal ventricle. The laryngeal ventricle contains mucous glands that lubricate the true cords, thus it is an important site for potential pathologic lesions.

SPECIFIC CONDITIONS
Reinke Edema

Background
Reinke edema, or polypoid corditis, is an accumulation of viscous material in the superficial lamina propria (Reinke space) of the true vocal cords. It is due to the chronic irritation of smoking.

Key features
Reinke edema is found most commonly in middle-aged women with a heavy smoking history. They complain of "sounding like a man" due to a low-pitched, raspy voice. On laryngoscopy, their vocal folds appear symmetrically edematous. During phonation, the cords look floppy.

Management
Reinke edema is at least partially reversible with smoking cessation. Surgical approaches do not necessarily provide full return of voice function and the problem recurs if the patient continues to smoke.

Laryngopharyngeal Reflux (LPR)

Background
LPR, also known as reflux laryngitis, is the term for laryngitis caused by irritation from reflux of gastric contents on the vocal cords and surrounding structures. It is related to gastroesophageal reflux disease (GERD) but the most patients do not have classic GERD symptoms. As many as half of patients who have laryngeal and voice disorders also have LPR.[4]

Key features
The most common symptoms of LPR are hoarseness, globus sensation, dysphagia, cough, chronic throat clearing, and sore throat.[4] Diagnosis is based on findings via laryngoscopy. The classic finding is evidence of inflammation on the posterior larynx, including edema, erosions, and/or granuloma formation (**Fig. 2**). Double-probe pH monitoring of the esophagus and pharynx simultaneously is the gold standard for diagnosis in questionable cases.[4]

Management
Proton pump inhibitors (PPIs) are customarily prescribed to treat LPR; however, a meta-analysis of eight randomized controlled trials demonstrated no better than modest benefit.[5] Treatment of LPR must be more aggressive and prolonged than

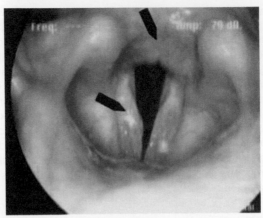

Fig. 2. Laryngopharyngeal reflux. The *arrows* point to edema in the posterior aspects of the larynx. (*From* Dworkin JP. Laryngitis: types, causes, and treatments. Otolaryngol Clin North Am 2008;41(2):419–36; with permission.)

for GERD because the larynx is more susceptible to reflux injury than the esophagus. This means twice daily PPI administration for 6 months or longer, though patients often experience symptom improvement within 2 to 3 months.[4] Symptom monitoring can be achieved with a validated nine-item questionnaire for office use.[6] When prolonged, aggressive PPI treatment fails, fundoplication is an effective treatment.[4]

Vocal Cord Nodules

Background

Vocal cord nodules are small, sessile, white masses symmetrically located on the edge of the midportion of each of the true vocal cords (**Fig. 3**). The midportion of the membranous vocal folds is the location of greatest impact between the vibrating cords, corresponding to their cause, vocal abuse. Incidence is highest in boys and middle-aged women.[7]

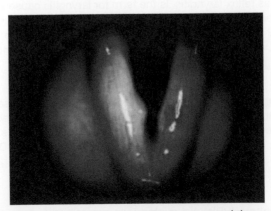

Fig. 3. Vocal cord nodules. (*From* Dhillon R, East CA. Ear, nose and throat and head and neck surgery: an illustrated color text. 4th edition. Philadelphia: Churchill Livingstone; 2013; with permission.)

Key features

Hoarseness is the most frequent initial symptom. Smoking does not seem to be an important etiologic factor.[7] Nodules are distinguished from polyps on laryngoscopy by their symmetry and more posterior location than polyps.

Management

Voice therapy is the initial treatment of vocal cord nodules; surgical excision is reserved for treatment failures.[8] Voice therapy involves three categories. The most effective method is physiologic, which optimizes voice production. The hygienic method, which improves behaviors that can lead to vocal cord injury, is of mixed benefit per systematic review. Symptomatic treatment of the abnormal voice quality has weak support.[9]

Vocal Cord Polyps

Background

Vocal fold polyps are a common, benign cause of hoarseness. They are usually unilateral and located at the free edge of the true vocal cord at the junction of the anterior and middle third (**Fig. 4**). They result from vocal abuse through a cyclic process of hematoma and/or separation of epithelial layers followed by inflammatory hyperplasia resulting in further voice strain and recurrent inflammatory response or fluid accumulation. Thus, they may appear red, white, or translucent, and may be broad-based or pedunculated.

Key features

Vocal cord polyps are distinguished from nodules by their asymmetry, more anterior location, and fleshy appearance. Inflammation in response to the primary lesion can develop into a contact lesion on the opposing vocal cord. Polyps are more common in men and are associated with vocal abuse but not with smoking.[7]

Management

Standard treatment of vocal cord polyps is surgical removal or laser ablation. However, in more than 50% of cases, hemorrhagic polyps may resolve with voice rest and voice therapy, so this is a reasonable alternative for patients who are willing to wait several months.[10]

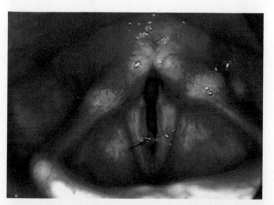

Fig. 4. Vocal cord polyp in right vocal fold (*arrow*). (*From* Martins RH, Defaveri J, Domingues MA, et al. Vocal polyps: clinical, morphologic, and immunohistochemical aspects. J Voice 2011;25(1):98–106; with permission of The Voice Foundation.)

Papillomas

Background

Human papillomavirus (HPV), primarily types 6 and 11, can cause recurrent warts on the vocal cords. Malignant transformation occurs in less than 2% of patients, so the primary morbidity for most patients is the propensity to recur, which requires repeated ablation procedures.[11] The exception is HPV type 16, which does show a propensity to develop into cancer. Whether HPV vaccination decreases the incidence of oropharyngeal cancer or of neonatal papillomatosis has not been demonstrated.[12]

Key features

Respiratory papillomatosis is the second most common cause of hoarseness in children. Papillomas should also be suspected in young adults with hoarseness, a group for which this complaint is otherwise less common than in older adults. On laryngoscopy, the lesions typically have a cauliflower-like exophytic appearance (**Fig. 5**).

Management

Because respiratory papillomatosis may be very aggressive in young children, especially those younger than 3 years old, early referral is indicated. The disease may require repeated surgeries, including tracheostomy, and can lead to death from respiratory failure.[13]

Treatment is microsurgery, with or without one of several laser options, in an effort to completely remove the papillomas yet preserve normal tissues. Antiviral chemotherapy is reserved for resistant or severe recurrent cases.[11]

Laryngeal Dysplasia and Cancer

Background

Nearly all laryngeal cancer is squamous cell carcinoma. The progression of the disease from precancer to cancer can be traced in the classification system from the World Health Organization: squamous cell hyperplasia, mild dysplasia, moderate dysplasia, severe dysplasia, carcinoma in situ, and invasive carcinoma.[14]

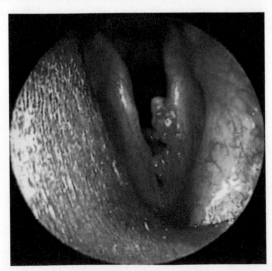

Fig. 5. Laryngeal papillomas. (*From* García JJ, Richardson MS. Common lesions of the larynx and hypopharynx. Surg Pathol Clin 2011;4(4):1153–75; with permission.)

The natural history of laryngeal cancer varies by location. Supraglottic tumors account for 30% to 35% of cancer cases. The supraglottic region has a rich lymphatic network that crosses the midline. In more than 50% of these patients, it has spread into regional lymph nodes at the time of diagnosis, resulting in more severe treatment approaches and worse prognosis than other locations. Tumors in the glottic region are present in 60% to 65% of patients. Here, the lymphatic drainage is sparse, so patients often present with less advanced disease and cure rates are 80% to 90%. Tumors of the subglottic region make up only 5% of laryngeal cancer cases.[12]

Key features
Most laryngeal carcinoma seems to be associated with tobacco and alcohol use, thus it is more common in men. Other potential associations to consider from the patient's history include HPV (see earlier discussion), occupational exposure to irritants, and LPR.[15] The primary lesion identified on laryngoscopy is leukoplakia that may or may not be accompanied by neovascularity or ulceration (**Figs. 6** and **7**).

Management
Visual evaluation does not correlate well with the severity of the dysplasia, so early referral for biopsy is recommended. The rate of progression of mild dysplasia to invasive cancer varies from 0% to 11.5%, so a protocol of regular follow-up is usually followed. Higher grades of dysplasia warrant immediate intervention.[3] The specific intervention of choice is a developing field of options that includes radiotherapy, microsurgery, and laser surgery techniques in an effort to preserve voice quality as much as possible while adequately removing or destroying the dysplastic lesions. All modalities can make it difficult for patients to eat adequate calories, so nutritional support and dietician involvement in care is important for decreasing the severity of weight loss during treatment.[12]

Following referral to subspecialists for cancer treatment, the primary physician can continue to play a key role in supportive care. Patients may assume that a diagnosis of laryngeal cancer means it is too late to stop smoking or cut back on alcohol consumption. However, these interventions may improve the efficacy of treatment and improve overall health outcomes, so they are worth pursuing.[12] In addition, patients often have

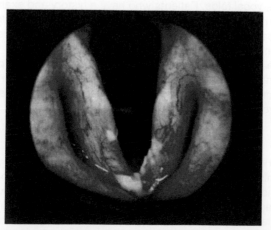

Fig. 6. Laryngeal leukoplakia. (*From* Benjamin B. Diagnostic laryngology: adults and children. Philadelphia: W.B. Saunders; 1989; with permission.)

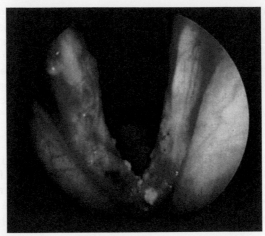

Fig. 7. Laryngeal carcinoma. (*From* Benjamin B. Diagnostic laryngology: adults and children. Philadelphia: W.B. Saunders; 1989; with permission.)

serious comorbidities related to their smoking and alcohol that require ongoing management.

Other Conditions

Asymmetric movement of the vocal cords signals injury of the recurrent laryngeal nerve. If there is no history of trauma to account for the finding, the possibility of thyroid cancer or metastatic lung cancer should be entertained.

Candidiasis of the hypopharynx and larynx can develop in immune-suppressed patients and patients on chronic or recurrent antibiotics or steroid inhalers. Typically, lesions are white plaques similar to those seen with candidiasis on other mucosal surfaces. Treatment is with clotrimazole troches or oral fluconazole.

Allergic rhinitis can cause hoarseness through several mechanisms. Nasal drainage can irritate the vocal cords. Allergens can exert a direct effect on the laryngeal mucosa. Finally, the antihistamines and decongestants used to treat allergies can dry the mucosa of the vocal folds. Patients who have a history and examination compatible with allergic rhinitis, commonly have findings of diffuse pale edema of the laryngeal mucosa. Treatment with topical nasal steroids avoids the side effects of other allergy medications.

Finally, hoarseness can be caused by a variety of neurologic and psychogenic dysphonias. On laryngoscopy, the operator may note symmetric changes of the vocal cords during functional assessment without anatomic lesions. Treatment is specific to the voice disorder.

SUMMARY

Patients commonly present to the primary care office with laryngeal complaints, particularly chronic hoarseness and cough. Most have benign conditions that can be diagnosed and treated without referral, including laryngopharyngeal reflux, the most common diagnosis. However, laryngeal carcinoma affects a small but significant portion of patients, especially smokers. Because early diagnosis and treatment are key elements to improving outcomes, patients should be evaluated with timely visualization of the larynx via nasolaryngoscopy.

REFERENCES

1. O'Sullivan BP, Finger L, Zwerdling RG. Use of nasopharyngoscopy in the evaluation of children with noisy breathing. Chest 2004;125:1265–9.
2. Golub JS, Chen PH, Otto KJ, et al. Prevalence of perceived dysphonia in a geriatric population. J Am Geriatr Soc 2006;54:1736–9.
3. Sadri M, McMahon J, Parker A. Management of laryngeal dysplasia: a review. Eur Arch Otorhinolaryngol 2006;263:843–52.
4. Koufman JA, Aviv JE, Shaw GY. Laryngopharyngeal reflux: position statement of the Committee on Speech, Voice, and Swallowing Disorders of the American Academy of Otolaryngology-Head and Neck Surgery. Otolaryngol Head Neck Surg 2002;127:32–5.
5. Qadeer MA, Phillips CO, Lopez AR, et al. Proton pump inhibitor therapy for suspected GERD-related chronic laryngitis: a meta-analysis of randomized controlled trials. Am J Gastroenterol 2006;101:2646–54.
6. Belafsky PC, Postma GN, Koufman JA. Validity and reliability of the reflux symptom index (RSI). J Voice 2002;16(2):274–7.
7. Nagata K, Kurita S, Yasumoto S, et al. Vocal fold polyps and nodules. A 10-year review of 1,156 patients. Auris Nasus Larynx 1983;10(Suppl):S27–35 [Tokyo].
8. Sulica L, Behrman A. Management of benign vocal fold lesions: a survey of current opinion and practice. Ann Otol Rhinol Laryngol 2003;112:827–33.
9. Thomas LB, Stemple JC. Voice therapy: does science support the art? Commun Dis Rev 2007;1(1):49–77.
10. Klein AM, Lehmann M, Hapner ER, et al. Spontaneous resolution of hemorrhagic polyps of the true vocal fold. J Voice 2009;23(1):132–5.
11. Derkay CS, Wiatrak B. Recurrent respiratory papillomatosis: a review. Laryngoscope 2008;118:1236.
12. National Comprehensive Cancer Network Guidelines Version 1. 2012. Head and Neck Cancers. Available at: http://www.nccn.org/professionals/physician_gls/f_guidelines.asp#site. Accessed May 6, 2013.
13. Morgan AH, Zitsch RP. Recurrent respiratory papillomatosis in children: a retrospective study of management and complications. Ear Nose Throat J 1986;65:19–28.
14. Barnes L, Eveson JW, Reichard P, et al. Pathology and genetics of head and neck tumours. WHO classification of tumours. Lyon (France): IARCS Press; 2005. p. 140–3.
15. Mau T. Diagnostic evaluation and management of hoarseness. Med Clin North Am 2010;94(5):945–60.

Nasolaryngoscopy

Scott E. Moser, MD

KEYWORDS

- Laryngopharyngeal reflux • Larynx • Endoscopy • Hoarseness • Vocal cord

KEY POINTS

- Nasolaryngoscopy is a low-risk, quick means of making a specific diagnosis for voice complaints.
- Nasolaryngoscopy should be performed before empiric treatment based on history and general examination alone.
- The most common indications for nasolaryngoscopy are hoarseness, globus sensation, and chronic cough.
- The most common findings from nasolaryngoscopy in a primary care setting include laryngopharyngeal reflux (43%), chronic rhinitis (32%), and vocal cord lesions (13%).

INTRODUCTION: NATURE OF THE PROBLEM

Hoarseness, chronic cough, globus sensation, and other nasolyngeal complaints are common reasons for patients to present to a family physician. Laryngeal carcinoma is also common, especially in smokers. There are no established guidelines for laryngeal cancer screening, but early diagnosis with definitive surgical treatment is important to survival.[1] The most common benign causes of nasolaryngeal complaints, such as chronic rhinitis and laryngopharyngeal reflux, are readily treatable by primary physicians. All these can be diagnosed safely and quickly with nasolaryngoscopy. For all these reasons, nasolaryngoscopy should be performed before empiric treatment based on history and general examination alone.[2] Alternative terms include nasopharyngoscopy and rhinolaryngoscopy.

Diagnostic nasolaryngoscopy is an easily mastered skill. The scope is simpler to operate than gastrointestinal endoscopes. The procedure is performed with only topical anesthesia, is well tolerated by patients, rarely causes complications, and can typically be performed in less than 10 minutes.

In addition to the anatomy of the laryngeal structures addressed previously, nasolaryngoscopy requires an understanding of the nasopharygeal anatomy the operator will encounter en route. This is also important, because nasolaryngoscopy can be used to evaluate a variety of nasal, sinus, and pharyngeal problems in addition to those of the larynx.

Department of Family and Community Medicine, University of Kansas School of Medicine-Wichita, 1010 North Kansas, Wichita, KS 67214, USA
E-mail address: smoser@kumc.edu

Prim Care Clin Office Pract 41 (2014) 109–113
http://dx.doi.org/10.1016/j.pop.2013.10.009
0095-4543/14/$ – see front matter © 2014 Elsevier Inc. All rights reserved.
primarycare.theclinics.com

As noted in (**Fig. 1**), key anatomic landmarks in the nose include the vestibule, septum, turbinates and their associated meati, the sinus ostia, and the choana. Important pharyngeal structures include the eustachian tube orifice surrounded by the torus tubarius and Rosenmüller fossa, the adenoid pad, and the palatine tonsils.

INDICATIONS/CONTRAINDICATIONS

The standard list of indications for nasolaryngoscopy is lengthy (**Box 1**), but the most common indications in a primary care setting are hoarseness (51%), globus sensation (32%), and chronic cough (17%).[3] Contraindications are few and straightforward, as noted in **Box 1**.

EQUIPMENT

Several manufacturers make excellent nasolaryngoscopes. Most are available in high-resolution video versions that cost more but offer advantages for instructing learners, allowing patients to see pathology for themselves, and capturing photos for documentation of findings. Some nasolaryngoscopes can use the same light source and video equipment with other scopes, minimizing the cost. The decision about which equipment to purchase should be based on both features and local support for staff training and equipment maintenance.

PATIENT PREPARATION

As with any procedure, the operator must obtain informed consent after careful discussion of indications, contraindications, anticipated benefits, risks, and alternatives.

The patient is seated upright or in a semi-supine position, most easily managed with a standard otolaryngology table, although an office examination table can also be used. The patient should be comfortable with foot support if necessary. Many patients enjoy being able to watch the procedure for themselves on the video monitor, so the operator should ask the patient's preference and position the patient and monitor accordingly. In addition, patients should be given tissues and a basin in case they experience sneezing or coughing.

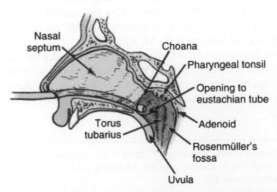

Fig. 1. Anatomic landmarks of the nose and pharynx. (*From* Fowler GC, Montalvo RO. Nasolaryngoscopy. In: Pfenninger JL, Fowler GC, editors. Pfenninger and Fowler's procedures for primary care. 3rd edition. Philadelphia: Saunders; 2011; with permission.)

> **Box 1**
> **Indications and contraindications for nasolaryngoscopy**
>
> Indications:
>
> Persistent hoarseness (>3 weeks)
>
> Chronic sinusitis or sinus discomfort, especially unilateral
>
> Suspected foreign body
>
> Suspected neoplasia
>
> Nasal polyps
>
> Chronic cough
>
> Chronic postnasal drip
>
> Recurrent epistaxis
>
> Recurrent otalgia
>
> Hemoptysis
>
> Dysphagia
>
> Head and neck masses
>
> Nasal obstruction or pain
>
> Chronic bad breath
>
> History of previous head and neck cancer
>
> Chronic rhinorrhea
>
> Recurrent or chronic serous otitis media in an adult
>
> Contraindications:
>
> Uncontrolled bleeding disorder
>
> Unable or unwilling to cooperate (eg, too young)
>
> Acute epiglottitis
>
> Acute epistaxis
>
> Recent facial trauma or surgery

TECHNIQUE

First, the operator determines which of the nares to enter with the nasolaryngoscope. This should be the symptomatic side for nasal problems and the most patent side for laryngeal problems. To determine the most patent side, the operator may occlude 1 nostril at a time with his or her gloved hand and instruct the patient to inhale through his or her nose. The quietest side is the most patent.

Commonly, the operator then applies a combination of topical decongestant to open the nasal passage and reduce the chance of bleeding and a topical anesthetic for comfort, including reduction of the risk of patient gagging. The need for these agents has been questioned in a meta-analysis of 8 randomized controlled trials.[4] A variety of techniques may be used. One common method is to allow the patient to spray oxymetazoline, 0.05% decongestant spray (Afrin), 2 to 3 puffs himself or herself from a standard 1 oz plastic mist bottle. Then the operator uses an atomizer to spray 2 or 4% plain lidocaine solution into the nose, making sure to direct the spray in several directions, including the nasal floor, the septum, and the spheno-ethmoidal recess. An alternative is to partly empty the oxymetazoline bottle and add lidocaine to it in a 1:1 ratio as a single combined application.[5] Topical cocaine can achieve both decongestion and anesthesia in a single application, but keeping such a controlled substance available in the office setting is problematic.

While waiting a couple of minutes for the anesthetic to take effect, the operator makes sure the scope and video equipment are operating properly and lenses are clean. The scope is more delicate than intestinal endoscopes, so gentle handling is critical. The scope is designed for the controls to be handled with the left hand and the tip with the right. The scope is directed up and down with the control knob and side to side by gentle twisting of the entire scope.

The operator rests the right hand on the patient's cheek in tripod fashion, controlling the scope tip with thumb and index finger, and inserts the tip into the nasal fossa, advancing it under direct vision to just above the epiglottis. Encouraging the patient to breathe through the nose facilitates soft palate movement away from the pharyngeal wall for a better view. If the scope fogs over, it can by cleared by instructing the patient to swallow. Similar to other endoscopic procedures, the focus during entry is on following the lumen with more careful examination as the scope is withdrawn. The operator should keep the tip of the scope above the level of the epiglottis and vocal cords in order to avoid laryngospasm. While viewing the cords, the patient is instructed through several maneuvers to observe cord function. When the patient says "E-E-E-E," both cords should come together symmetrically. When the patient whispers, only the anterior portion of the cords should approximate symmetrically. The vallecula can be evaluated by asking the patient to stick out his or her tongue.

After viewing laryngeal structures, the operator withdraws the scope to view pharyngeal and nasal structures. Palate and eustachian tube function can be evaluated with, "key- key- key." The area around the eustachian tube orifice should be observed on both right and left, paying special attention to Rosenmüller fossa, an important potential site for carcinoma. As the scope tip reaches the choana, the operator directs it superiorly to view the sphenoid recess. The maneuver can cause the patient to sneeze, so it should be performed gently and quickly. As the scope is further withdrawn, the superior and middle meati are evaluated, including visualization of various sinus ostia for pus or polyps. Finally, the scope is straightened to remove.

COMPLICATIONS AND MANAGEMENT

Complications are rare and usually minor, such as blood pressure elevation, sneezing or gagging severe enough to limit the procedure, and vasovagal reaction. Potentially serious risks include: adverse reaction to the decongestant or anesthetic, laryngospasm, vomiting with potential aspiration, and bleeding secondary to injury.

POSTOPERATIVE CARE

Patients should be instructed to take nothing by mouth until they sense the anesthetic has worn off, usually less than 1 hour. Then they should try sips of water. If patients tolerate sips without difficulty, they can return to normal diet and activity.

REPORTING, FOLLOW-UP, AND CLINICAL IMPLICATIONS

Because the procedure is performed under local anesthesia, the operator should discuss findings with the patient immediately and negotiate the next steps of the plan. As with any diagnostic procedure, a brief note explaining the final diagnosis and plan handed to the patient on exit is a good idea. The operator should immediately and carefully annotate the procedure, findings, and plan in the patient's medical record. The scope should be cleaned and dried per manufacturer's recommendations.

OUTCOMES

The most common findings from nasolaryngoscopy in a primary care setting include laryngopharyngeal reflux (43%), chronic rhinitis (32%), and vocal cord lesions (13%). More than 1% of patients in 1 study were discovered to have laryngeal cancer.[3] The high prevalence of carcinoma and benign treatable conditions reinforces the value of this procedure in primary care.

CURRENT CONTROVERSIES/FUTURE CONSIDERATIONS

Stoboscopy, adding variable speed strobe lighting while viewing the vocal folds, offers the opportunity to more accurately assess function of the cords as they vibrate. This feature improves diagnostic accuracy by as much as 47% in subtle cases but is not considered standard of care for routine evaluation of hoarseness. It should be considered anytime the patient's symptoms seem out of proportion to the findings on standard nasolaryngoscopy.[2]

SUMMARY

Nasolaryngoscopy is a low-risk, quick means of making a specific diagnosis for voice complaints. Because most laryngeal problems are benign and treatable without referral, and because early diagnosis and treatment are important for laryngeal carcinoma, nasolaryngoscopy should be performed before empiric treatment based on history and general examination alone. Under topical anesthesia, the scope is inserted through the nose and advanced to directly view the larynx. During withdrawal, structures of the pharynx and nose are also evaluated. Complications are rare and usually minor.

REFERENCES

1. Sadri M, McMahon J, Parker A. Management of laryngeal dysplasia: a review. Eur Arch Otorhinolaryngol 2006;263:843–52.
2. Schwartz SR, Cohen SM, Dailey SH, et al. Clinical practice guideling: hoarseness (dyphonia). Otolaryngol Head Neck Surg 2009;141:S1–31.
3. Wilkins T, Gillies RA, Getz A, et al. Nasolaryngoscopy in a family medicine clinic: indications, findings, and economics. J Am Board Fam Med 2010;23(5):591–7.
4. Conlin AE, McLean L. Systematic review and meta-analysis assessing the effectiveness of local anesthetic, vasoconstrictive, and lubricating agents in flexible fibre-optic nasolaryngoscopy. J Otolaryngol Head Neck Surg 2008;37(2):240–9.
5. Strauss RA. Flexible endoscopic nasopharyngoscopy. Atlas Oral Maxillofac Surg Clin North Am 2007;15:111–28.

Dizziness and Vertigo

Jennifer Wipperman, MD, MPH

KEYWORDS

- Benign paroxysmal peripheral vertigo • Vestibular neuritis • Vestibular migraine
- Meniere's disease • Migrainous vertigo • Acute labyrinthitis

KEY POINTS

- Benign paroxysmal peripheral vertigo (BPPV) is the most common cause of vertigo. It is diagnosed using the Dix-Hallpike maneuver and treated with the Epley maneuver.
- Vestibular neuritis is a single episode of acute, severe vertigo. The head thrust test and visual fixation can help differentiate it from acute stroke. The mainstay of treatment is vestibular rehabilitation.
- Vestibular migraine manifests as vertigo accompanied by classic migraine symptoms, and responds to migraine medications.
- Over eighty percent of patients with Meniere's disease can be successfully managed with lifestyle changes and diuretics.

INTRODUCTION

Dizziness is a common and challenging condition seen in the primary care office. More than one-third of Americans see a health care provider for dizziness during their lifetime.[1] Although most dizziness is due to benign causes, life-threatening causes, such as a stroke or intracranial mass, also need to be excluded. Because "dizziness" is a vague term that can include a wide array of medical disorders, it is important to use a stepwise approach to differentiate between causes.

First, clinicians should distinguish between the four common types of dizziness: (1) presyncope, (2) disequilibrium, (3) psychogenic dizziness, and (4) vertigo. Patients should be asked to specifically describe their dizziness in their own words. Vertigo is a false sense of motion of either the environment or self. Often, patients describe a feeling of the room spinning or tilting. Benign paroxysmal peripheral vertigo (BPPV), vestibular neuritis, vestibular migraine, and Meniere's disease are the four most common causes of vertigo in ambulatory settings, and a thorough history and physical examination alone can lead to the diagnosis in most cases (**Table 1**).

BENIGN PAROXYSMAL PERIPHERAL VERTIGO

BPPV is the most common cause of vertigo. Patients typically report brief episodes triggered by head movement. A positive Dix-Hallpike maneuver is diagnostic, and

Department of Family and Community Medicine, University of Kansas School of Medicine - Wichita, 1010 North Kansas, Wichita, KS 67214, USA
E-mail address: jennifer.wipperman@viachristi.org

Table 1
Characteristics of common causes of vertigo

	BPPV	Vestibular Neuritis	Vestibular Migraine	Meniere's Disease
Time Course	Recurrent, lasting seconds	Single episode lasting days	Recurrent, lasting minutes to days	Recurrent, lasting hours
History	Brief, triggered by head movement	Subacute onset of severe, constant vertigo with significant nausea and vomiting	Previous history of migraine. Vertigo accompanied by migraine symptoms	Hearing loss, tinnitus and ear fullness
Nystagmus	Up-beating torsional	Horizontal or horizontal-torsional	Usually none	Horizontal or horizontal-torsional
Gait	Normal	Veers toward affected side	Abnormal during vertigo attacks	May have impaired gait and imbalance
Auditory Symptoms	None	Hearing loss (acute labyrinthitis)	None	Present
Diagnostic Findings	Positive Dix-Hallpike maneuver	Positive head-thrust test, Nystagmus suppressed by visual fixation	Vertigo attacks resolve with acute migraine medications	Repeat audiometry shows fluctuating, low-frequency hearing loss

canalith repositioning procedures (CRP), such as the Epley maneuver, are the mainstay of treatment.

Epidemiology

BPPV accounts for more than 40% of vertigo diagnoses seen in primary care, and is the most common cause of vertigo across the lifespan.[2] Patients with BPPV most commonly present between the fifth and seventh decades of life, and it is seen more commonly in women.[3] By 80 years of age, nearly 10% of adults have been diagnosed with BPPV during their lifetime.[4]

Risk Factors

A history of prior head trauma or prior vestibular disorders, such as vestibular neuritis, increases a patient's risk of BPPV. Osteoporosis and vitamin D deficiency have been associated with BPPV.[5] Recently, sleep position has also been correlated with BPPV, with patients who have BPPV being more likely to report lying on their sides with the affected ear down.[6]

Pathophysiology

It is hypothesized that BPPV is caused by loose calcium carbonate debris (otoconia) in the semicircular canals of the inner ear. With head motion, otoconia begin to move freely in the canals. When head motion stops, otoconia continue to move, causing endolymph to move against the hair cells of the semicircular canal. This leads to a false sense of motion that lasts until the otoconia settle, usually only a few seconds. The posterior canal is involved in 85% of cases, followed by the horizontal canal in 10% of cases.[7] Rarely, BPPV can be bilateral.

Clinical Presentation

In BPPV, patients complain of brief episodes of vertigo triggered by position changes. Episodes usually last only seconds, and are less than 1 minute in duration. Commonly, patients experience attacks when rolling over in bed, or tilting the head to look upward. Patients may report difficulty placing objects on high shelves, or bending forward to tie shoes. Nausea and vomiting may occur with episodes. Vertigo from most causes is exacerbated by certain movements. In BPPV, however, vertigo is actually *preceded* by position changes and patients are normal between attacks.

Physical examination should include a complete ear, nose, and throat, cardiovascular, and neurologic evaluation. This is to exclude other causes of vertigo (**Table 2**), because there are no specific physical examination findings in BPPV. However, the Dix- Hallpike and supine roll tests are two maneuvers that can confirm BPPV suspected by historical clues.

Diagnosis

The diagnosis of BPPV is made clinically. It is confirmed most often with the Dix-Hallpike maneuver, and in some cases the supine roll test.

Diagnostic maneuvers

The Dix-Hallpike maneuver should be performed in any patient being evaluated for BPPV (**Fig. 1**). It is used to diagnose posterior canal BPPV. Before performing the Dix-Hallpike, clinicians should warn patients that severe vertigo, and possibly nausea, may occur. Patients sit upright on an examination table with the head rotated 45 degrees to the right. Maintaining this head position, the examiner quickly lays the patient back into the supine position, and extends the neck approximately 20 degrees so that the head "hangs" supported off the edge of the examination table. The examiner then observes the patient for vertigo and nystagmus. In posterior canal BPPV, nystagmus is up-beating and torsional. Characteristically, there is a latency period of 5 to 20 seconds after the position change to the onset of nystagmus and vertigo. The nystagmus and vertigo initially increase in intensity and then resolve within 60 seconds ("crescendo-decrescendo" nystagmus). The side that provokes symptoms indicates the involved ear. Even if positive, the Dix-Hallpike should be repeated on the opposite side to exclude bilateral BPPV. A positive Dix-Hallpike test requires observation of the characteristic nystagmus. If a persistent or down-beating nystagmus is elicited, a central cause should be suspected.

If the Dix-Hallpike maneuver is negative, a supine roll test should be performed to diagnose lateral canal BPPV (**Fig. 2**). For the supine roll test, the patient begins in the

Table 2	
Differential diagnosis of vertigo	
Peripheral Causes	**Central Causes**
BPPV	Migrainous vertigo
Vestibular neuritis	Intracranial mass
Meniere's disease	Cerebrovascular attack
Perilymphatic fistula	Vertebrobasilar insufficiency
Herpes zoster oticus	Chiari malformation
Acoustic neuroma	Multiple sclerosis
Ototoxicity	Episodic ataxia type 2
Otitis media	
Semicircular canal dehiscence syndrome	
Posttraumatic vertigo (labyrinth concussion)	

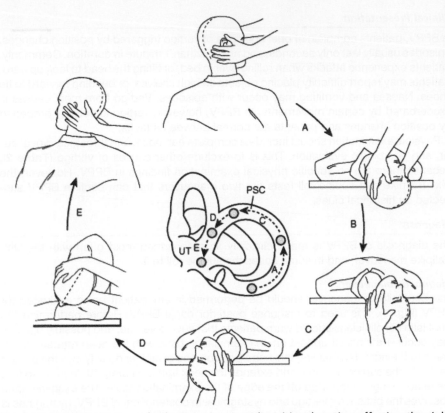

Fig. 1. Treatment maneuver for benign paroxysmal positional vertigo affecting the right ear. To treat the left ear, the procedure is reversed. The drawing of the labyrinth in the center shows the position of the particle as it moves around the posterior semicircular canal (PSC) and into the utricle (UT). The patient is seated upright, with head facing the examiner, who is standing on the right. (A) The patient is rapidly moved to head-hanging right position (Dix-Hallpike test). This position is maintained until the nystagmus ceases. (B) The examiner moves to the head of the table, repositioning hands as shown. (C) The head is rotated quickly to the left with right ear upward. This position is maintained for 30 seconds. (D) The patient rolls onto the left side while the examiner rapidly rotates the head leftward until the nose is directed toward the floor. This position is then held for 30 seconds. (E) The patient is rapidly lifted into the sitting position, now facing left. The entire sequence should be repeated until no nystagmus can be elicited. After the maneuver, the patient is instructed to avoid head-hanging positions to prevent the particles from reentering the posterior canal. (*From* Rakel RE. Conn's current therapy 1995. Philadelphia: WB Saunders; 1995. p. 839; with permission.)

supine position with their head facing upward. The examiner quickly moves the patient's head 90 degrees to one side, and examines for nystagmus and vertigo. The supine roll test should be repeated to the opposite side. In lateral canal BPPV, nystagmus is most often a geotrophic type: horizontal and beating toward the lower (affected) ear during the supine roll test. When rolled to the opposite side, the nystagmus recurs and beats toward the lower (unaffected) ear but is less intense. Less often, nystagmus may be of apogeotrophic type: horizontal and beating toward the upper ear.

If the Dix-Hallpike and supine roll tests are negative, another diagnosis should be suspected. However, if the clinical history is strongly indicative of BPPV, then the

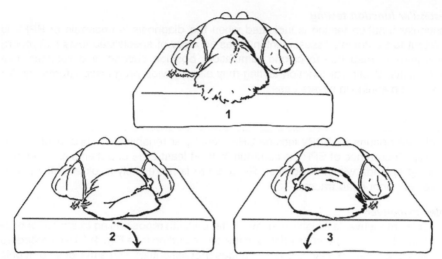

Fig. 2. Supine roll test. (1) Start supine with head in neutral position. (2) Turn the patient's head quickly 90 degrees to the right and observe for nystagmus. Return the head to neutral position (1). (3) After any residual nystagmus or symptoms resolve, turn the patient's head quickly 90 degrees to the left and observe for nystagmus. (*From* Fife TD, Iverson DJ, Lempert T, et al. Practice parameter: therapies for benign paroxysmal positional vertigo (an evidence-based review): report of the Quality Standards Subcommittee of the American Academy of Neurology. Neurology 2008;70:2067–74; with permission.)

patient should return in 1 week to repeat the maneuvers. Although the positive predictive value of the Dix-Hallpike maneuver is 83%, its negative predictive value is 52%.[2] Therefore, it is worth repeating to avoid a false-negative result.

Radiographic imaging
Patients with BPPV do not require neuroimaging unless the diagnosis is uncertain and a central cause is suspected (**Table 3**). Magnetic resonance imaging (MRI) is the best imaging test in most cases because it includes the posterior fossa, and is useful for evaluating central causes, such as a cerebrovascular lesion, intracranial mass, or demyelinating disease.

Table 3 Red flags for a central cause
History
Sudden onset New, severe headache Cardiovascular risk factors
Nystagmus
Direction-changing Purely vertical or torsional Unsuppressed by visual fixation
Inability to walk
Negative head-thrust test
Additional neurologic signs (e.g. aphasia, dysarthria, weakness, sensory loss)

Vestibular function testing

Vestibular function testing is indicated when the diagnosis is uncertain or BPPV is resistant to treatment. Assessment involves an array of specialized tests that record nystagmus in response to caloric stimulation, position change, and voluntary eye movements. Vestibular function testing may also provide prognostic information for treatment planning in severe cases.

Treatment

Treatment options for BPPV include CRP, vestibular rehabilitation, observation, and surgery. Recurrence of BPPV is common, with at least 25% of patients experiencing a repeat episode within 6 months.[8] Recurrence is more likely in older patients and those with prior head trauma.

Epley maneuver

The Epley maneuver is a highly effective, safe, canalith repositioning treatment of posterior canal BPPV that can be offered in the office setting (see **Fig. 1**).[7] This procedure consists of a series of head position changes that essentially settle the loose otoconia from the semicircular canal into the utricle, where they can no longer trigger vertigo attacks. The Epley maneuver is effective in more than 90% of cases, and has an odds ratio of 4.2 (95% confidence interval, 2.0–9.1) for symptom resolution.[9] Patients who suffered severe nausea or vomiting with the Dix-Hallpike may require pretreatment with an antiemetic. The liberatory (Semont) maneuver can be tried for patients who cannot physically undergo the Epley maneuver. Postural restrictions, such maintaining upright posture and limiting cervical motion, may add a slight benefit to CRP alone.[10] Home CRP exercises are also effective, and may be especially useful for expedient self-treatment if future episodes recur.[11]

Lempert maneuver

The Lempert maneuver (barbeque roll maneuver) treats lateral canal BPPV.[12] Lying supine, the patient is rolled 90 degrees and held until symptoms stop. This is continued for a full 360 degrees. Interestingly, a case report also noted successful treatment of lateral canal BPPV with repeated somersaults.[13]

Vestibular rehabilitation

Vestibular rehabilitation is a series of physical therapy exercises that improve central compensation for a peripheral deficit causing vertigo. Exercises usually consist of moving the head while eyes are fixed on an object, or moving the body while moving the head. Although less effective than CRP in the short-term, vestibular exercises are more effective than observation, and reach similar effectiveness rates to CRP by 3 months' follow-up.[14] Furthermore, vestibular rehabilitation may prevent recurrence of BPPV, especially in the elderly.

Pharmacologic

Treatment with vestibular-suppressant medications, such as benzodiazepines and antihistamines, should be avoided in BPPV. These medications can blunt central compensation, and increase risk of falls. Furthermore, there is no evidence that treatment of BPPV with vestibular-suppressant medications is effective.[7]

Observation

Because BPPV can remit spontaneously, usually over the course of 4 to 6 weeks, observation is a potential treatment option. Observation may be considered for patients with mild BPPV, or those who may not tolerate CRP or vestibular rehabilitation.

However, patients are at higher risk of falls until BPPV resolves and recurrence is more likely.

Surgical treatment

Surgery is rarely indicated, and is reserved for severe, refractory cases of BPPV. Surgically occluding the posterior canal with a plug is effective in 90% of cases, with 5% experiencing permanent hearing loss.[15] Other surgical options include laser ossification of the posterior canal and posterior ampullary nerve transection.

VESTIBULAR NEURITIS

Vestibular neuritis is an acute, prolonged attack of severe vertigo that is thought to be of viral origin. Symptomatic care is the mainstay of treatment, because most cases resolve spontaneously with complete recovery. Although a benign disorder, it must be differentiated from more serious causes of acute vertigo, such as a cerebrovascular accident.

Epidemiology

Vestibular neuritis is the second most common cause of vertigo. It accounts for almost 10% of all patients seen for dizziness.[16] Most patients diagnosed are 30 to 50 years of age. Men and women are affected equally. There are no well-studied risk factors for vestibular neuritis.

Pathophysiology

Vestibular neuritis is thought to be caused by a viral infection of the eighth cranial nerve. Supporting evidence includes an increased incidence of vestibular neuritis during viral epidemics, and the common precedence of vestibular neuritis by a viral syndrome. Herpes simplex virus may be an etiologic agent, because studies have identified herpes simplex virus-1 DNA in the vestibular ganglia of patients with vestibular neuritis.[17] Viral infection may lead to inflammation, and potentially atrophy, of the vestibular nerve causing severe vertigo.

Clinical Presentation

Vertigo is sudden in onset, persistent, and severe. Patients may report awakening with severe vertigo, or may experience a subacute onset, with vertigo worsening over several hours. Vertigo is most severe for the first 1 to 2 days, and then gradually improves over several weeks. Initially, patients may have significant nausea and vomiting. Any motion worsens the vertigo; therefore, many may prefer to lie still with their eyes closed.

On physical examination, patients have a spontaneous nystagmus at the onset of illness. The nystagmus is unidirectional and horizontal/horizontal-torsional, with the fast phase beating away from the affected side. The nystagmus can be suppressed by visual fixation. Visual fixation can be tested by asking the patient to focus on an object in the room (nystagmus ceases) and then placing a blank sheet of paper in front of the patient's face (nystagmus resumes). Importantly, a central lesion, such as acute stroke, often presents with spontaneous nystagmus unsuppressed by visual fixation.

When assessing gait, patients with vestibular neuritis tend to veer toward the affected side. An inability to walk, however, is a red flag for a central cause. Hearing is normal in vestibular neuritis. When hearing loss is associated, the condition is known as acute labyrinthitis. Other neurologic signs and symptoms are not found in vestibular neuritis; their presence should raise concern for a central cause.

Diagnosis

Like BPPV, the diagnosis of vestibular neuritis is made clinically. Specialized physical examination maneuvers, such as the head-thrust test, can help differentiate between vestibular neuritis and a more concerning central lesion, such as acute stroke.

Head-thrust test

The head-thrust test is a useful maneuver to differentiate vestibular neuritis from a central cause (**Fig. 3**). The head-thrust test is performed by quickly moving the patient's head 10 degrees to the right and left while the patient's eyes remain fixed on the examiner's nose. If a saccade (patient's eyes move briefly off target) is present, then the test is positive for a peripheral lesion. Central vertigo does not exhibit a saccade.

HINTS: three steps to rule out stroke

The head-impulse-nystagmus-test-of-skew (HINTS) is a combination of three clinical signs that can be tested in patients with acute vertigo to differentiate between

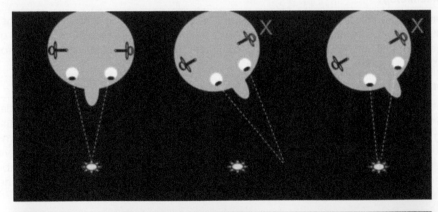

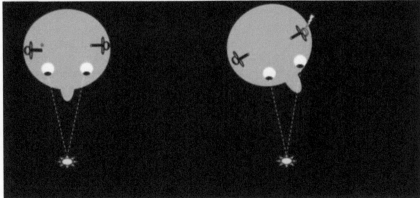

Fig. 3. Head-thrust test. *Top panel* shows a positive head-thrust test. The examiner moves the patient's head quickly 10 degrees to the side, in this case to the patient's left. A catch-up saccade is observed when the patient looks away and then refixes on the visual target, indicating a peripheral lesion on the left. *Bottom panel* shows a normal head-thrust test. The patient maintains visual fixation during head movement. (*From* Seemungal BM, Bronstein AM. A practical approach to acute vertigo. Pract Neurol 2008;8:211–21; with permission.)

vestibular neuritis and stroke. These signs include the head-thrust test, nystagmus, and skew deviation. Nystagmus that is bidirectional, purely vertical, or purely torsional is concerning for stroke. Skew deviation (supranuclear vertical eye misalignment, or vertical strabismus) is assessed with the cover/uncover test. Any patient with one or more of these signs should be evaluated for stroke. Using HINTS, stroke can be detected with 100% sensitivity and 96% sensitivity.[18]

Radiographic imaging
Neuroimaging, such as MRI, is reserved for patients with additional risk factors for stroke, additional neurologic signs, severe headache, or as needed to rule out a suspected central lesion based on clinical findings.

Vestibular function testing
Vestibular testing may be useful if the diagnosis is unclear. In vestibular neuritis, testing demonstrates a unilateral vestibular loss.

Treatment

Symptomatic care and vestibular rehabilitation are the mainstays of treatment in vestibular neuritis. Although some endorse systemic corticosteroids, there is currently insufficient evidence for routine use.[19] Antiviral medications are ineffective.[20]

Medications
Initially, vertigo and associated nausea and vomiting can be treated with a combination of antihistamine (dimenhydrinate [Dramamine], 50 mg every 6 hours), antiemetic (promethazine [Phenergan], 25 mg every 6 hours), and benzodiazepine (lorazepam [Ativan], 1–2 mg every 4 hours) medications. Patients with severe symptoms may need to be hospitalized for intravenous fluids and medications. Medications should be discontinued after 2 to 3 days because of their vestibular-suppressant effect. Initial recovery in vestibular neuritis is because of central compensation, followed later by the return of vestibular function. Vestibular suppressants can block central compensation and thus impede resolution if used for prolonged periods.

Vestibular rehabilitation
As opposed to medications, vestibular exercises hasten recovery in vestibular neuritis. Exercises increase central compensation for the peripheral defect, thereby improving balance, ocular stability, gait, and vertigo. Compared with placebo, vestibular rehabilitation has an odds ratio of 2.67 (95% confidence interval, 1.85–3.86) for symptom improvement.[14] Patients should begin exercises as soon as the acute phase resolves and movement is tolerable, generally within 2 to 3 days of onset. Exercises may be home-based or formally supervised.

VESTIBULAR MIGRAINE

Vestibular migraine is often an unrecognized cause of episodic vertigo. Patients usually have other migraine symptoms with attacks, such as headache and photophobia, which differentiate it from other causes of vertigo. Treatment is similar to other types of migraine headache.

Epidemiology

Vestibular migraine is a common cause of recurrent, episodic vertigo, but is underrecognized. It is 5 to 10 times more common than Meniere's disease, and approximately 1% of the population is affected at any time.[21,22] Vestibular migraine is more common among children than adults, with an estimated prevalence of nearly 3% among children aged 6 to 12 years.[23] Among adults, it is three times more common among women than men, and more often seen during the third to fifth decade of life.[21] Family history is a significant risk factor.

Pathophysiology

As a variant of migraine, vestibular migraine has a similar pathophysiology. Although not well-understood, it is theorized that migraine results from central vascular dysregulation and abnormal neuronal activity. Certain triggers may lead to vasoconstriction of the cerebrovasculature and hypoxia, and concurrent neuronal depolarization leads to aura and headache.[24] Other terms for vestibular migraine include migraine-associated vertigo and migrainous vertigo.

Clinical Presentation

As the name suggests, patients with vestibular migraine experience symptoms of vertigo and migraine. Although most patients experience vertigo close in timing with their migraine headaches, the two may not occur simultaneously. Vertigo may precede headache (like a vertiginous aura), coincide with headache, or occur separately. Vertigo can be spontaneous or triggered by position changes. Many patients experience head motion intolerance and visual vertigo (vertigo brought on by watching a moving object, such as traffic). Vertigo may last minutes, hours, or days. If patients do not experience headache with vertigo, then often there are other symptoms of migraine, such as aura, photophobia, or phonophobia. Often, vertigo episodes have similar triggers to migraines, such as lack of sleep, menstruation, and skipped meals. Most patients do not experience aural symptoms, such as hearing loss and tinnitus. Clues distinguishing vestibular migraine from Meniere's disease include an attack lasting days and normal hearing.

The physical examination is normal in patients with vestibular migraine, unless presenting during a vertigo attack. At that time, patients may exhibit signs of imbalance, such as a positive Romberg test.

Diagnosis

Vestibular migraine is a clinical diagnosis and one of exclusion. Diagnostic criteria have been developed that specify definite and probable vestibular migraine (**Box 1**).[25] A "dizzy diary" is helpful to identify symptoms and timing of vertigo in relation to headaches. If the diagnosis remains unclear, vertigo that responds to migraine medications suggests vestibular migraine. There is no confirmatory test for vestibular migraine; however, it is prudent to obtain audiometry and vestibular function tests to exclude other causes. Patients with migraine are more likely than the general population to have vestibular disorders, such as Meniere's disease and BPPV.[26,27]

Treatment

There is little evidence to guide treatment of vestibular migraine, and recommendations are mostly based on expert opinion.[21] However, following principles of migraine management, most patients can attain good control of vertigo.

Lifestyle
Patients should identify and avoid triggers for their vertigo or migraines. Regular sleep, meals, and exercise benefit most patients.

Box 1
Diagnostic criteria for vestibular migraine

Definite vestibular migraine

A. Episodic vestibular symptoms of at least moderate severity

B. Current or previous history of migraine according to the 2004 criteria of the International Headache Society (IHS)

C. One of the following migrainous symptoms during two or more attacks of vertigo: migrainous headache, photophobia, phonophobia, visual aura, or other aura

D. Other causes excluded

Probable vestibular migraine

A. Episodic vestibular symptoms of at least moderate severity

B. One of the following: (1) current or previous history of migraine according to the 2004 IHS criteria; (2) migrainous symptoms during vestibular symptoms; (3) migraine precipitants of vertigo in more than 50% of attacks (food triggers, sleep irregularities, or hormonal change); or (4) response to migraine medications in more than 50% of attacks

C. Other causes excluded

Medications

For vertigo, vestibular suppressants noted previously, such as dimenhydrinate, promethazine, and meclizine (Antivert, 25 mg every 8 hours) can be helpful. Acute vertigo can be aborted with triptans as used for migraine. Patients with frequent, severe, or prolonged episodes should be offered migraine-prophylactic medications. Preventive medications include β-blockers, anticonvulsants, tricyclic antidepressants, and calcium channel blockers. A reasonable goal is to reduce the frequency of attacks by 50%.

Vestibular rehabilitation

For patients with chronic imbalance or vertigo, vestibular exercises may be considered.

MENIERE'S DISEASE

The triad of episodic vertigo, fluctuating hearing loss, and tinnitus is the hallmark of Meniere's disease. Because of its remitting and relapsing nature, the diagnosis is challenging. However, most patients can be reassured that vertigo can be significantly controlled with lifestyle changes and medication.

Epidemiology

The incidence and prevalence of Meniere's disease is difficult to determine because of its periodic nature. However, its estimated prevalence is 0.2%, with women slightly more affected than men.[28] There is a genetic preponderance of Meniere's; other risk factors include a prior history of vestibular neuritis, head trauma, and syphilic otitis.[29]

Pathophysiology

Endolymphatic hydrops is presumed to be the underlying cause of Meniere's.[30] Dysregulation of fluid results in swelling in the endolymphatic compartment, leading to symptoms of vertigo, hearing loss, tinnitus, and aural pressure. Eventually, swelling may cause permanent damage to vestibular structures. There are multiple potential causes of endolymphatic hydrops, including genetic, autoimmune, vascular, viral, allergic, and traumatic.[31] Meniere's disease is the term for the idiopathic form. When a cause is identified (prior trauma, syphilic otitis) it is termed Meniere's syndrome.

Clinical Presentation

The classic symptoms of Meniere's disease include vertigo, hearing loss, tinnitus, and aural fullness. Symptoms tend to vary widely among patients. Some patients mainly experience aural symptoms, some mainly vertigo, and others may be equally affected.

Vertigo attacks are acute in onset and severe. Episodes usually last a few hours, but are at least 20 minutes in duration and can last up to 24 hours. Vertigo attacks are often preceded by aural fullness or tinnitus. Vertigo may be described as a spinning or rocking sensation, and may be associated with nausea and vomiting. In some patients, attacks may cluster over a period of a few weeks, whereas others can experience years of remission. Over time, patients may experience positional vertigo or general imbalance between episodes because of progressive loss of vestibular function.

Hearing loss in Meniere's disease is fluctuating (usually in relation to vertigo episodes but may be separate), initially in the low frequencies (**Fig. 4**). As the disease progresses hearing loss becomes permanent and involves all frequencies. Tinnitus is usually described as a roaring sensation, and tends to change pitch and loudness during vertigo attacks. Patients often experience a feeling of fullness or pressure in the involved ear associated with hearing loss.

Otolithic crises of Tumarkin are sudden, random drop attacks that patients with Meniere's may experience. There is no associated loss of consciousness, but their unpredictable nature places patients at risk of serious trauma. Therefore, patients with Tumarkin crises should be aggressively treated.

On physical examination, patients with Meniere's disease may have notable hearing loss and potentially balance or gait difficulty depending on the severity of the disease

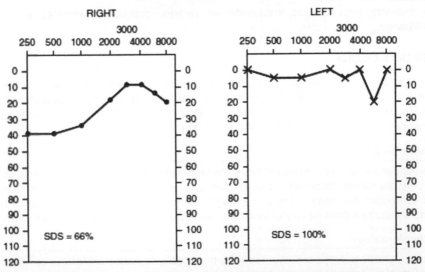

Fig. 4. Audiogram of low-frequency hearing loss in Meniere's disease. SDS, speech discrimination score. (*From* Bope ET, Kellerman RD. Conn's Current Therapy 2013. Philadelphia: Saunders; 2012. p. 301; with permission.)

or if presenting during a vertiginous attack. With vertigo episodes, patients manifest a unidirectional, horizontal-torsional nystagmus. Although there may be no physical examination findings in a patient with Meniere's disease, a complete physical examination is crucial to exclude other causes.

Diagnosis

Currently, the diagnosis of Meniere's disease is made clinically because there is no specific diagnostic test for the disease. Diagnostic criteria are listed in **Box 2**. For a definite diagnosis, patients must have had at least two episodes of vertigo lasting at least 20 minutes, audiometrically documented hearing loss on at least one occasion, and tinnitus or aural fullness in the affected ear.[32] Successive audiograms showing fluctuating hearing loss are very helpful, especially if obtained during attacks of vertigo.

Radiographic imaging
MRI is usually obtained to exclude other causes of vertigo and hearing loss, such as acoustic neuroma, aneurysms, or multiple sclerosis.

Vestibular function testing
Vestibular testing is not necessary for diagnosis, but may be useful for determining bilaterality of disease and candidates for interventional treatments. Initially, testing may be normal, but with progressive disease most patients show vestibular hypofunction on caloric testing. The vestibular evoked myogenic potential is a newer method used for diagnosis and monitoring, but has not yet been fully validated.[33]

Box 2
Diagnostic criteria for Meniere's disease

Certain Meniere's disease

   Definite Meniere's disease plus histopathologic confirmation

Definite Meniere's disease

A. ≥2 definitive spontaneous episodes of vertigo 20 min or longer

B. Audiometrically documented hearing loss on at least 1 occasion

C. Tinnitus or aural fullness in the treated ear

D. Other causes excluded

Probable Meniere's disease

A. One definitive episode of vertigo

B. Audiometrically documented hearing loss on at least 1 occasion

C. Tinnitus or aural fullness in the treated ear

D. Other causes excluded

Possible Meniere's disease

A. Episodic vertigo without documented hearing loss, or Sensorineural hearing loss fluctuating or fixed, with disequilibrium but non-episodic

B. Other causes excluded

Adapted from Committee on hearing and equilibrium guidelines for the diagnosis and evaluation of therapy in Meniere's disease. American Academy of Otolaryngology-Head and Neck Foundation, Inc. Otolaryngol Head Neck Surg 1995;113(3):181–5; with permission.

Treatment

Goals of treatment are to decrease the frequency and severity of vertigo, improve balance, preserve hearing, and improve overall quality of life. Patients should be educated that Meniere's is a chronic condition with no cure, but that with treatment nearly all patients have significant improvement of vertigo. Unfortunately, hearing loss and tinnitus are more difficult to control. Treatment uses a stepwise approach, starting with lifestyle changes and adding diuretics if necessary. Eight percent of patients attain control of vertigo with conservative treatment.[34] If medical management fails, several interventional options are available.

Lifestyle changes

Many patients can achieve adequate control of symptoms with dietary changes and avoidance of triggers. Episodes can be precipitated by high salt intake, caffeine, alcohol, allergies, nicotine, monosodium glutamate, and stress. Patients should limit salt intake to less than 2 g daily, and limit caffeine and alcohol to one drink daily. Treatment of allergies, including immunotherapy, can significantly improve symptoms.[35]

Medications

Vestibular-suppressant medications are useful during acute attacks of vertigo. An oral steroid burst is often given as well, although evidence for its efficacy is limited and it is being replaced by intratympanic steroid injection.[36]

If lifestyle changes do not effectively control vertigo, then daily diuretics may be added. A typical regimen is triamterene-hydrochlorothiazide (Dyazide), 37.5 to 25 mg daily, although other diuretics may be used. Betahistine (Serc) is a vasodilator and antihistamine commonly used in Europe for prophylaxis, but it is not available within the United States.[37]

Vestibular rehabilitation

Vestibular exercises may be beneficial for patients who experience imbalance or disequilibrium between attacks of vertigo, and for the elderly to reduce falls.[14]

Hearing aids

Patients with bilateral hearing loss can benefit from hearing aids. However, because of the fluctuating nature of hearing loss, many patients become frustrated with hearing aids.

Intratympanic glucocorticoids

Injection of glucocorticoid into the middle ear through the tympanic membrane can improve vertigo in many patients. Although less effective than other treatments, it is minimally invasive and has the potential to improve hearing.[36] Approximately 40% of patients achieve complete control of vertigo with intratympanic glucocorticoid injections.[38,39] One trial conducted over 2 years found that 90% of patients had adequate control of vertigo with repeated steroid injection, obviating the need for more invasive treatment.[40]

Meniett device

The Meniett device is a portable machine that delivers pulses of positive pressure to the middle ear through a tympanostomy tube. Theoretically, this controls symptoms by improving endolymphatic drainage. Although there is limited evidence that the Meniett device is effective, it only requires placement of a tympanostomy tube and does not cause hearing loss.[41]

Endolymphatic sac procedures
Endolymphatic sac procedures involve drainage of endolymphatic fluid by placing a shunt to the mastoid and/or decompression. There is some controversy regarding the effectiveness of the procedures, but there is minimal risk of hearing loss and reports of long-term effectiveness in 75% of patients.[15,42] This procedure is generally indicated for patients who have failed prior medical treatment and wish to preserve hearing.

Intratympanic gentamycin
Gentamycin is an aminoglycoside antibiotic that is vestibulotoxic and cochleotoxic. Intratympanic gentamycin causes a "chemical labyrinthectomy" when injected through the middle ear to be absorbed by the inner ear. Studies report more than 95% effectiveness; however, up to one-third of patients have permanent hearing loss.[43,44] Therefore, it is often reserved for treatment of patients with intractable vertigo and significant hearing loss.

Vestibular neurectomy
Severing the vestibular nerve is the most definitive treatment for controlling vertigo when the goal is to preserve hearing, achieving control in 95% of patients.[45] However, neurectomy requires general anesthesia, a craniotomy, and overnight monitoring in an intensive care unit. It also has several potential risks, such as facial nerve damage.

Labyrinthectomy
Surgical destruction of the labyrinth is a highly effective method for eliminating vertigo, but also causes irreversible hearing loss. It is therefore reserved for patients with intractable vertigo who have failed other treatments and have no serviceable hearing in the involved ear.[31]

Bilateral disease
Bilateral Meniere's disease affects approximately 15% of patients. However, over time it is estimated that up to 30% or more develop disease in both ears.[46] Bilateral Meniere's disease presents a treatment challenge. Treating one side may not relieve vertigo, and interventional treatment can cause permanent hearing loss in a patient already at risk of hearing loss in both ears.

SUMMARY

Vertigo is a common problem that often brings patients into the primary care office. BPPV, vestibular neuritis, vestibular migraine, and Meniere's disease are the four most common causes of vertigo. Because these conditions are mainly diagnosed based on clinical grounds, clinicians should be familiar with their history, physical examination findings, and diagnostic criteria. With this armament, primary care physicians should feel well-equipped to aid the dizzy patient.

REFERENCES

1. Agrawal Y, Carey JP, Della Santina CC, et al. Disorders of balance and vestibular function in US adults: data from the National Health and Nutrition Examination Survey, 2001-2004. Arch Intern Med 2009;169(10):938–44.
2. Hanley K, O' Dowd T. Symptoms of vertigo in general practice: a prospective study of diagnosis. Br J Gen Pract 2002;52(483):809–12.
3. Neuhauser HK. Epidemiology of vertigo. Curr Opin Neurol 2007;20(1):40–6.

4. von Brevern M, Radtke A, Lezius F, et al. Epidemiology of benign paroxysmal positional vertigo: a population based study. J Neurol Neurosurg Psychiatr 2007; 78(7):710–5.
5. Buki B, Ecker M, Junger H, et al. Vitamin D deficiency and benign paroxysmal positioning vertigo. Med Hypotheses 2013;80(2):201–4.
6. Shigeno K, Ogita H, Funabiki K. Benign paroxysmal positional vertigo and head position during sleep. J Vestib Res 2012;22(4):197–203.
7. Bhattacharyya N, Baugh RF, Orvidas L, et al. Clinical practice guideline: benign paroxysmal positional vertigo. Otolaryngol Head Neck Surg 2008;139(5 Suppl 4): S47–81.
8. Perez P, Franco V, Cuesta P, et al. Recurrence of benign paroxysmal positional vertigo. Otol Neurotol 2012;33(3):437–43.
9. Hilton M, Pinder D. The Epley (canalith repositioning) manoeuvre for benign paroxysmal positional vertigo. Cochrane Database Syst Rev 2004;(2):CD003162.
10. Hunt WT, Zimmermann EF, Hilton MP. Modifications of the Epley (canalith repositioning) manoeuvre for posterior canal benign paroxysmal positional vertigo (BPPV). Cochrane Database Syst Rev 2012;(4):CD008675.
11. Cohen HS, Sangi-Haghpeykar H. Canalith repositioning variations for benign paroxysmal positional vertigo. Otolaryngol Head Neck Surg 2010;143(3): 405–12.
12. Fife TD, Iverson DJ, Lempert T, et al. Practice parameter: therapies for benign paroxysmal positional vertigo (an evidence-based review): report of the Quality Standards Subcommittee of the American Academy of Neurology. Neurology 2008;70(22):2067–74.
13. Czesnik D, Liebetanz D. Granddaughter's somersault treats cupulolithiasis of the horizontal semicircular canal. Am J Otol 2013;34(1):72–4.
14. Hillier SL, McDonnell M. Vestibular rehabilitation for unilateral peripheral vestibular dysfunction. Cochrane Database Syst Rev 2011;(2):CD005397.
15. Sismanis A. Surgical management of common peripheral vestibular diseases. Curr Opin Otolaryngol Head Neck Surg 2010;18(5):431–5.
16. Neuhauser HK, Lempert T. Vertigo: epidemiologic aspects. Semin Neurol 2009; 29(5):473–81.
17. Arbusow V, Theil D, Strupp M, et al. HSV-1 not only in human vestibular ganglia but also in the vestibular labyrinth. Audiol Neurootol 2001;6(5):259–62.
18. Kattah JC, Talkad AV, Wang DZ, et al. HINTS to diagnose stroke in the acute vestibular syndrome: three-step bedside oculomotor examination more sensitive than early MRI diffusion-weighted imaging. Stroke 2009;40(11):3504–10.
19. Fishman JM, Burgess C, Waddell A. Corticosteroids for the treatment of idiopathic acute vestibular dysfunction (vestibular neuritis). Cochrane Database Syst Rev 2011;(5):CD008607.
20. Strupp M, Zingler VC, Arbusow V, et al. Methylprednisolone, valacyclovir, or the combination for vestibular neuritis. N Engl J Med 2004;351(4):354–61.
21. Cherchi M, Hain TC. Migraine-associated vertigo. Otolaryngol Clin North Am 2011;44(2):367–75, viii–ix.
22. Neuhauser HK, Radtke A, von Brevern M, et al. Migrainous vertigo: prevalence and impact on quality of life. Neurology 2006;67(6):1028–33.
23. Abu-Arafeh I, Russell G. Paroxysmal vertigo as a migraine equivalent in children: a population-based study. Cephalalgia 1995;15(1):22–5 [discussion: 24].
24. Neuhauser H, Lempert T. Vestibular migraine. Neurol Clin 2009;27(2):379–91.
25. Neuhauser H, Lempert T. Vertigo and dizziness related to migraine: a diagnostic challenge. Cephalalgia 2004;24(2):83–91.

26. Radtke A, Lempert T, Gresty MA, et al. Migraine and Meniere's disease: is there a link? Neurology 2002;59(11):1700–4.
27. Ishiyama A, Jacobson KM, Baloh RW. Migraine and benign positional vertigo. Ann Otol Rhinol Laryngol 2000;109(4):377–80.
28. Alexander TH, Harris JP. Current epidemiology of Meniere's syndrome. Otolaryngol Clin North Am 2010;43(5):965–70.
29. Sajjadi H, Paparella MM. Meniere's disease. Lancet 2008;372(9636):406–14.
30. Nakashima T, Naganawa S, Sugiura M, et al. Visualization of endolymphatic hydrops in patients with Meniere's disease. Laryngoscope 2007;117(3):415–20.
31. Semaan MT, Megerian CA. Meniere's disease: a challenging and relentless disorder. Otolaryngol Clin North Am 2011;44(2):383–403, ix.
32. Committee on Hearing and Equilibrium guidelines for the diagnosis and evaluation of therapy in Meniere's disease. American Academy of Otolaryngology-Head and Neck Foundation, Inc. Otolaryngol Head Neck Surg 1995;113(3):181–5.
33. Taylor RL, Wijewardene AA, Gibson WP, et al. The vestibular evoked-potential profile of Meniere's disease. Clin Neurophysiol 2011;122(6):1256–63.
34. Santos PM, Hall RA, Snyder JM, et al. Diuretic and diet effect on Meniere's disease evaluated by the 1985 Committee on Hearing and Equilibrium guidelines. Otolaryngol Head Neck Surg 1993;109(4):680–9.
35. Derebery MJ. Allergic and immunologic features of Meniere's disease. Otolaryngol Clin North Am 2011;44(3):655–66, ix.
36. Hamid M. Medical management of common peripheral vestibular diseases. Curr Opin Otolaryngol Head Neck Surg 2010;18(5):407–12.
37. Lacour M, van de Heyning PH, Novotny M, et al. Betahistine in the treatment of Meniere's disease. Neuropsychiatr Dis Treat 2007;3(4):429–40.
38. Casani AP, Piaggi P, Cerchiai N, et al. Intratympanic treatment of intractable unilateral Meniere's disease: gentamicin or dexamethasone? A randomized controlled trial. Otolaryngol Head Neck Surg 2012;146(3):430–7.
39. Barrs DM, Keyser JS, Stallworth C, et al. Intratympanic steroid injections for intractable Meniere's disease. Laryngoscope 2001;111(12):2100–4.
40. Boleas-Aguirre MS, Lin FR, Della Santina CC, et al. Longitudinal results with intratympanic dexamethasone in the treatment of Meniere's disease. Otol Neurotol 2008;29(1):33–8.
41. Gurkov R, Filipe Mingas LB, Rader T, et al. Effect of transtympanic low-pressure therapy in patients with unilateral Meniere's disease unresponsive to betahistine: a randomised, placebo-controlled, double-blinded, clinical trial. J Laryngol Otol 2012;126(4):356–62.
42. Wetmore SJ. Endolymphatic sac surgery for Meniere's disease: long-term results after primary and revision surgery. Arch Otolaryngol Head Neck Surg 2008; 134(11):1144–8.
43. Pullens B, van Benthem PP. Intratympanic gentamicin for Meniere's disease or syndrome. Cochrane Database Syst Rev 2011;(3):CD008234.
44. Huon LK, Fang TY, Wang PC. Outcomes of intratympanic gentamicin injection to treat Meniere's disease. Otol Neurotol 2012;33(5):706–14.
45. Li CS, Lai JT. Evaluation of retrosigmoid vestibular neurectomy for intractable vertigo in Meniere's disease: an interdisciplinary review. Acta Neurochir 2008;150(7): 655–61 [discussion: 661].
46. Nabi S, Parnes LS. Bilateral Meniere's disease. Curr Opin Otolaryngol Head Neck Surg 2009;17(5):356–62.

Neurologic Syndromes of the Head and Neck

John N. Dorsch, MD

KEYWORDS

- Facial nerve paralysis • Trigeminal neuralgia • Herpes zoster

KEY POINTS

- Malignant (necrotizing) otitis externa can cause facial paralysis in addition to ear pain. Ear pain from necrotizing otitis externa is described as severe, deep, constant pain. If facial nerve paralysis is present, eye care with artificial tears in the day time, lubricating ointment at night time, and taping the eyelid shut at night should be done to protect against corneal abrasion and ulceration.
- Herpes zoster (HZ) can occur along the distribution of any nerve after reactivation of varicella zoster, including the cranial nerves.
- Treatment of HZ oticus consists of combined antiviral and corticosteroid therapy. About 75% of patients of HZ oticus will recover from facial paralysis provided treatment is begun within the first 72 hours of onset of symptoms. Early diagnosis is therefore critical.
- Bell's palsy is a term for *idiopathic* facial nerve paralysis, although it is now widely believed that reactivation of Herpes Simplex Virus type 1 (HSV-1) accounts for most Bell's palsy cases. Some cases of Bell's palsy may be attributed to ischemia and microvascular disease from diabetes mellitus, analogous to diabetic mononeuropathy. Bell's palsy is believed to account for 60% to 75% of all cases of unilateral facial paralysis.
- Facial paralysis in children is different than in adults in that up to 70% of cases have identifiable secondary causes compared to 25% to 40% in adults. Except in areas endemic for Lyme disease, the most common cause of facial paralysis in children is acute otitis media.
- A patient experiencing a trigeminal neuralgia paroxysm typically freezes in place with hands slowly rising to the area of pain on the face but not touching it. He or she then grimaces with an involuntary spasm of the facial muscles referred to as tic douloureux and then either remains in this position or cries out in pain.

Although patients with Bell's palsy and trigeminal neuralgia occasionally present to primary care physicians, most of the syndromes in this article are somewhat rare in primary care practice. It is important to recognize signs and symptoms of these syndromes so that appropriate management is carried out. Patients may experience sensory (pain, neuralgia, altered taste, hypesthesia, altered hearing, etc.) and/or motor

Funding Sources: Nil.
Conflict of Interest: Nil.
Department of Family & Community Medicine, University of Kansas School of Medicine - Wichita, 1010 North Kansas, Wichita, KS 67214, USA
E-mail address: jdorsch@kumc.edu

Prim Care Clin Office Pract 41 (2014) 133–149
http://dx.doi.org/10.1016/j.pop.2013.10.012

(paresis/paralysis) symptoms of the head and neck due to disorders of the cranial and cervical nerves. The syndromes and symptoms discussed in this article include ear pain, sinus pain, herpes zoster (HZ) oticus (Ramsay Hunt), HZ ophthalmicus, facial nerve paralysis in adults and children, superior laryngeal neuralgia, trigeminal neuralgia, glossopharyngeal neuralgia, nervus intermedius (geniculate) neuralgia, and Raeder paratrigeminal syndrome.

EAR PAIN

The ear is innervated by sensory fibers from cranial nerves V, VII, IX, and X, as well as the second and third cervical nerves.[1] When ear pain is caused by intrinsic ear disease, such as otitis media or otitis external, the otologic examination is usually abnormal. Common causes of ear pain with a normal ear examination include neuralgias and referred pain from conditions such as temporomandibular joint disorders, pharyngitis, dental disease, cervical spine arthritis, and neuralgias.

There are many causes of ear pain.[1] **Table 1** lists causes of ear pain and their distinguishing characteristics. A focused history, physical examination, and diagnostic testing will help differentiate these causes (**Box 1**).

Malignant (necrotizing) otitis externa can cause facial paralysis in addition to ear pain.[2] Ear pain from necrotizing otitis externa is described as severe, deep, constant pain. If facial nerve paralysis is present, eye care with artificial tears in the day time, lubricating ointment at night time, and taping the eyelid shut at night should be done to protect against corneal abrasion and ulceration.

Patients with ear pain not explained by otologic findings who have a significant history of tobacco or alcohol use and are older than 55 years of age should be considered for nasolaryngoscopy and enhanced MRI of the head and neck to look for tumors of the nose, nasopharynx, oral cavity, oropharynx, infratemporal fossa, and neck.[1] Other significant risk factors raising the suspicion of tumor include dysphagia, weight loss, radiation exposure, and hoarseness.

Patients with temporal (giant cell) arteritis typically experience temporal pain and tenderness that may occasionally radiate to the ear. They also commonly experience malaise, weight loss, fever, anorexia, and visual loss. Most patients with temporal arteritis have elevated erythrocyte sedimentation rates, and may or may not have a positive biopsy of the temporal artery.

SINUS PAIN

Sinus pain can be confused with facial pain from other sources, such as neuralgia. Acute purulent rhinosinusitis can cause both local and referred pain. These are the common patterns of pain referral:

- Maxillary sinusitis causes pain and tenderness over the cheek. Pain tends to be constant and burning in nature with zygomatic and dental tenderness.[3]
- Frontal sinusitis causes frontal (forehead) pain and tenderness.[4]
- Sphenoid and ethmoidal sinusitis causes pain behind and between the eyes.[4]

Pain from rhinosinusitis is typically exacerbated when the patient bends forward and relieved as soon as the infected material drains from the sinus.[4]

HERPES ZOSTER

HZ can occur along the distribution of any nerve after reactivation of varicella zoster, including the cranial nerves. The elderly and patients who have diminished

Table 1
Differential diagnosis of ear pain

Diagnosis	Distinguishing Characteristics
Otitis media	Abnormal examination of tympanic membrane
Otitis externa	Pain elicited by traction on ear; swelling and erythema of external auditory canal with debris
Foreign body	Visible on otoscopic examination
Barotrauma	TM hemorrhage and/or serous or hemorrhagic middle ear fluid; pain onset of airplane descent or while scuba diving
TMJ syndrome	Tender TMJ; crepitus of clicking with opening and closing mouth
Dental causes	Caries, abscesses, gingivitis, teeth tender to percussion
Pharyngitis	Erythema of throat, swelling, exudate, sore throat
Necrotizing (malignant) otitis externa	Associated with osteitis of the base of the skull, granulation tissue on floor of external auditory canal, may cause facial nerve palsy, older and immunocompromised patients, especially diabetics
HZ oticus	Vesicular rash on auricle, facial nerve paralysis, hearing loss, vertigo
Cellulitis/perichondritis	Preceding insect bite, piercing, scratch usually involving lobe
Relapsing polychondritis	Recurrent swelling and redness of auricle; a systemic disease involving cartilage but spares the earlobes (where there is no cartilage); often involves both ears
Trauma	Blunt or sharp, lacerations, frostbite
Mastoiditis	Recent or concurrent otitis media; pain behind ear
Tumors or cysts in auricle or canal	History of smoking, alcohol use, age >50, hoarseness, dysphagia, weight loss
Neuralgias	Brief attacks of pain that is intense, episodic, electric shocklike
Temporal arteritis	Older age, jaw claudication, vision loss, high ESR
Oral aphthous ulcers	Localized pain in mouth with sores
Cervical adenopathy	URI, tender cervical nodes
Eagle syndrome (elongated styloid)	Deep, pain exacerbated by swallowing or chewing
Sinusitis	Nasal congestion; tender over involved sinuses
Carotidynia	Dysphagia and throat tenderness; tender carotid artery; more common in women with migraine
Thyroiditis	Pain in thyroid with tenderness and referral to ear
Salivary gland disorders	Pain in front of ear, prominent and tender parotid glands
GERD	Acid reflux, heartburn; referral to ear
Angina pectoris	Cardiac risk factors
Thoracic aneurysms	Older men usually, chest or back pain
Psychogenic	History of depression or anxiety
Ramsay Hunt syndrome (HZ oticus)	HZ of cranial nerves VII and VII
Cholesteatoma	May be painful, but more likely associated with a sense of fullness of the ear
Tumors in the nose, nasopharynx, oropharynx, oral cavity, infratemporal fossa, neck, chest	May cause referred pain to the ear

Abbreviations: ESR, erythrocyte sedimentation rate; GERD, gastroesophageal reflux disease; TMJ, temporomandibular joint; URI, upper respiratory tract infection.

Adapted from Ely J, Hansen M, Clark E. Diagnosis of ear pain. Am Fam Physician 2008;77(5):621–8; with permission.

Box 1
Key history, physical testing, and diagnostic testing to differentiate causes of ear pain

History

- What is the location of pain? (Ask the patient to point to the pain with their finger).
- Does the pain radiate? If so, where?
- What aggravates the pain? (eg, chewing, swallowing, coughing)?
- Are the associated symptoms? (otologic or systemic)
- Are there risk factors for tumors (eg, age >50, tobacco and/or alcohol use)?
- Do symptoms favor a primary disorder of the ear (discharge, tinnitus, hearing loss, vertigo)?
- Is there a history of significant allergy or recent upper respiratory infection (eustachian tube dysfunction)?
- Has there been recent air travel, scuba diving history, or other causes of barotrauma?

Physical Examination

- Examine the auricle. Tenderness with traction on the auricle indicates otitis externa.
- Perform a thorough otoscopic examination (foreign body in ear canal, erythema of temporomandibular joint or ear canal)?
- Palpate temporomandibular joint for tenderness and crepitus as patient opens and closes mouth.
- Palpation of the head, face, and neck. Frontal, maxillary, sphenoid, and ethmoid sinusitis can cause referred pain.
- Inspect the nose and oropharynx.
- Inspect the gingiva and percuss the teeth with a tongue depressor to detect dental disease.
- Examine the cranial nerves.

Diagnostic tests

- Assessment of hearing.
- Pneumatic otoscopy or tympanometry to test mobility of tympanic membrane.
- Nasolaryngoscopy and enhanced magnetic resonance imaging (MRI) of the head and neck if patient is at high risk for tumor (MRI is best for soft tissue involvement).
- Computed tomography (CT) with contrast if MRI result is positive or if history of trauma to temporal bone (to look for bone involvement).

---

cell-mediated immunity (HIV, malignancy, immunosuppressive therapy, chemotherapy, corticosteroid use, and emotional stress) are more likely to develop HZ.[5] Typically, patients developing HZ have a prodrome of 2 to 3 days with varying degrees of pain. Descriptions of the quality of pain may include "burning, shooting, stabbing, or throbbing." After the prodrome, most patients develop a dermatomal rash that is initially erythematous, then papular, then vesicular. These lesions usually become pustular about 1 week after the rash begins. Late appearance of new vesicles beyond 1 week of rash onset often indicates an immunodeficiency syndrome.[5] Adjacent dermatomes may occasionally be involved. Disseminated HZ involving multiple dermatomes is more commonly seen in immunocompromised patients. Approximately 5% of patients with HZ will have a second episode; most of these patients are immunocompromised.[5] Post-herpetic neuralgia (PHN) is a common complication from HZ. PHN is defined as at least 90 continuous days of documented pain. The incidence of

PHN increases with age.[6] Sometimes pain can be evoked by stimuli that normally would not cause pain, such as light touch with a cotton swab. This is known as allodynia and is somewhat common in acute HZ pain, as well as PHN.

The treatment of HZ is with antiviral drugs. Acyclovir (800 mg 5 times a day for 7 days), valacyclovir (1000 mg 3 times a day for 7 days), or famciclovir (500 mg 3 times a day for 7 days) should be prescribed within 48 to 72 hours of onset of the rash.[5] Antiviral drugs do not, unfortunately, prevent or cure chronic pain from HZ. They also do not eradicate the virus. Antivirals are effective against viral replication, thus reducing the duration of viral shedding and new lesion formation. Antiviral drugs have been shown to decrease the duration and severity of acute pain of HZ.[5] By reduction of acute neural damage, antiviral drugs are believed to significantly reduce the duration of pain in PHN.[5] Corticosteroids given in the acute stages of HZ do not seem to prevent chronic pain of PHN, but they have been demonstrated to significantly reduce acute pain from HZ.[5] HZ vaccine should not be used in the treatment of HZ. Acute and chronic pain from HZ can be treated with tricyclic antidepressants, venlafaxine, duloxetine, opioids, tramadol, gabapentin, pregabalin, nerve blocks, and intravenous VZV hyperimmune globulin.[5]

HERPES ZOSTER OPHTHALMICUS

Patients with HZ ophthalmicus (HZO) typically have a prodrome of severe headache, malaise, and fever, with unilateral pain (or hypesthesia) in the affected eye and on the forehead and top of the head.[7] The distribution of HZO is the V1 (ophthalmic) distribution of the trigeminal nerve. Along with vesicular eruption of the dermatome, patients commonly have conjunctivitis, episcleritis, and drooping of the eyelid. When the rash spreads down the nose, indicating nasociliary branch involvement, viral keratitis occurs (Hutchinson sign).[8] Keratitis is typically a very painful condition that may appear as a corneal abrasion or as a branching ("dendritic") pattern on fluorescein staining of the cornea. HZO keratitis is a potentially sight-threatening condition. Patients with HZO should be referred to ophthalmologists urgently. Approximately two-thirds of patients with HZO are estimated to develop keratitis.[8]

HERPES ZOSTER OTICUS: RAMSAY HUNT SYNDROME

The incidence of HZ oticus (HZ otics) is 5 per 100,000 per year, mostly in patients older than 60 years of age.[9,10] **Box 2** lists the clinical characteristics of HZ oticus.

HZ oticus was first termed "HZ cephalicus" by James Ramsay Hunt,[11] who described varicella zoster virus (VZV) involvement of cranial nerves V, VII, VIII, IX, and X. HZ oticus is caused by reactivation of latent VZV in the geniculate ganglion and affects both cranial nerves VII and VIII due to their close proximity to one another.[5] Approximately 8% of patients with HZ oticus do not have vesicles, a condition known as "sine herpete."[12] Mucocutaneous vesicles may also occur in the oral mucosa or on the tongue.

Patients with facial nerve paralysis from HZ oticus tend to have a worse prognosis for recovery of facial muscle function than patients with Bell's palsy.[12] Recovery of facial function from HZ oticus is often incomplete, as is recovery of hearing and problems with balance. When patients have facial nerve paralysis with concomitant severe pain or sensorineural hearing loss, a diagnosis of HZ oticus should be considered instead of Bell's palsy.[11] Prediction for recovery of facial paralysis often cannot be made until 3 weeks after the onset of facial palsy. Electroneuronographic (ENG) studies of facial nerve function performed between days 10 and 14 for HZ oticus have been recommended by some experts, but may not routinely provide accurate information on the prognosis or recovery rate from facial paralysis.[13]

> **Box 2**
> **Clinical characteristics of HZ oticus**
>
> - Vesicles of the auricle or ear canal with ear pain
> - Facial paralysis
> - Tinnitus
> - Sensorineural hearing loss
> - Hyperacusis/dysacusis
> - Vertigo
> - Dysgeusia
>
> *Data from* Adour KK. Otological complications of Herpes Zoster. Ann Neurol 1994;35:S62–4.

Treatment of HZ oticus consists of combined antiviral and corticosteroid therapy. About 75% of patients of HZ oticus will recover from facial paralysis provided treatment is begun within the first 72 hours of onset of symptoms.[5,9] Early diagnosis is therefore critical. Antiviral treatment options include acyclovir (800 mg 5 times daily for 7–10 days), valacyclovir (1000 mg 3 times a day for 7–10 days), or famcyclovir (500 mg 3 times a day for 7–10 days).[9] One example of a common corticosteroid regimen is prednisone, 60 mg/d, for 14 days, then taper over 7 days.[14] Treatment with corticosteroids is believed to relieve acute pain, reduce vertigo, and speed healing of skin lesions.[14]

BELL'S PALSY AND OTHER CAUSES OF FACIAL PARALYSIS

The incidence of Bell's palsy is 20 to 30 cases per 100,000[15] per year. The highest incidence is in the 70s age group.[16] The gender distribution is equal,[15] and Bell's palsy is more common in diabetic and pregnant women.[17]

Bell's palsy is a term for *idiopathic* facial nerve paralysis, whereas it is now widely believed that reactivation of herpes simplex virus type 1 (HSV-1) accounts for most Bell's palsy cases.[18] Some cases of Bell's palsy may be attributed to ischemia and microvascular disease from diabetes mellitus, analogous to diabetic mononeuropathy.[16] Bell's palsy is believed to account for 60% to 75% of all cases of unilateral facial paralysis.[16] **Box 3** outlines the clinical presentation of Bell's palsy. Other causes of facial paralysis are numerous and are listed in **Table 2**.

The facial nerve (cranial nerve VII) supplies innervation to all the muscles of facial expression, parasympathetic fibers to the lacrimal and salivary glands, and sensory fibers for taste to the anterior two-thirds of the tongue.

Stroke and Bell's palsy are the 2 most common causes of *abrupt onset* of facial paralysis.[16] One study noted that most Bell's palsy patients first noticed their paralysis on awakening in the morning.[15] Patients first notice that they cannot close the affected eye and that water spills from the mouth when they try to drink. The study theorized that ischemia of facial nerve increases at night (causing edema of cranial nerve VII, entrapment of cranial nerve VII in the bony facial nerve canal, and reactivation of HSV-1 in the geniculate ganglion). Ischemic brain and heart disease incidence also appear to be increased at night.[15]

A familial tendency in Bell's palsy has been reported in 2.4% to 28.6% of cases.[19] Patients with familial Bell's palsy have *recurrences* of facial paralysis more often[20] and tend to have Bell's palsy at younger ages than other patients. A viral cause is not

> **Box 3**
> **The clinical presentation of Bell's palsy**
>
> - Weakness or complete paralysis of all the muscles on one side of the face
> - Disappearance of facial creases, nasolabial folds, and forehead furrows
> - Drooping of the corner of the mouth
> - Failure of the eyelids to close
> - Eye rolls upward on attempt to close the eyelid (Bell's phenomenon)
> - Eye irritation resulting from dryness to exposure and reduction of tear production
> - Food and saliva may pool in the affected side of the mouth and may spill out from the corner of the mouth
> - Preservation of facial sensation (although patients may have a perception of numbness from paralysis)
> - Hyperacusis from paralysis of stapedius muscles (paralysis results in no dampening of vibration of the ossicles, and sounds are abnormally loud on the affected side); there is no hearing loss from Bell's palsy[16]

implicated in familial Bell's palsy. Proposed causes of familial Bell's palsy include an inherited anatomic abnormality of the facial canal, vascular risk factors (eg, diabetes mellitus, hypertension), and other immunogenetic factors. Familial Bell's palsy appears to have an autosomal dominant pattern of inheritance.[19]

Progression of facial paralysis that is *slow or gradual in onset*, progressive in nature, and without evidence of spontaneous recovery should raise the suspicion of tumor as the cause of facial paralysis. Benign and malignant neoplasms are estimated to account for about 5% of all cases of peripheral facial nerve paralysis, with parotid carcinomas the most common.[21]

Four historical findings appear to be important in recommending surgical exploration of the facial nerve for tumor involvement:[22]

Table 2
Etiologies of facial paralysis

Category	Examples
Idiopathic	Bell's palsy
Congenital	Traumatic birth, Moebius syndrome, trisomies 13 and 18
Trauma	Basal skull fracture, penetrating injury to middle ear, barotrauma
Neurologic	Amyloidosis, multiple sclerosis
Metabolic	Pregnancy, diabetes mellitus, hypertension, hyperthyroidism
Neoplastic	Parotid tumors, cholesteatoma, glomus tumor, cranial nerve tumors, metastatic carcinomas, neurofibromatosis
Vascular	Anomalous or ectatic vessels, carotid artery aneurysm
Infection	Otitis externa, otitis media, mastoiditis, Lyme disease, numerous other infections
Iatrogenic	Mandibular block anesthesia, intranasal influenza vaccine, parotid surgery, mastoid surgery, dental procedures, post-immunization, post-T&A
Autoimmune	Temporal arteritis, Thrombotic thrombocytopenic purpura, Periarteritis nodosa, Guillain-Barré, multiple sclerosis, sarcoidosis

- Progressive and prolonged pattern of paralysis without recovery
- History of pain
- Involvement of other cranial nerves
- History of regional skin cancer

Imaging consisting of enhanced MRI and contrast-enhanced CT of the temporal bone, brain, neck, and parotid gland should be done when tumor is suspected. About 85% of patients with Bell's palsy have some degree of spontaneous recovery of facial function by 3 weeks.[17] One author has recommended that imaging should be considered if there is no spontaneous recovery of facial paralysis by 12 weeks and tumor is suspected.[21]

Evaluation of the patient with facial paralysis is summarized in **Box 4**.[17]

Patients with older age, hypertension, impairment of taste, pain other than in the ear, and complete facial weakness have a poorer prognosis for recovery of facial nerve function.[16] Corticosteroids are usually given for Bell's palsy. A common regimen is prednisone, 60 mg/d, tapering over 10 days.[17] Another proposed regimen is prednisone, 1 mg/kg daily, for 7 days, starting within 2 to 14 days after onset of symptoms.[16] One study showed significant improvement in the cure rate in diabetics when they were given intravenous prednisolone, 200 mg/d, for 2 days tapered to 70 mg by day 7.[25]

Antiviral drugs, given with corticosteroids, are believed to cause a slightly higher recovery rate than from corticosteroids alone.[16] Antiviral drug regimens studied include acyclovir, 400 mg 5 times per day, for 7 days and valacyclovir, 1 gm 3 times a day, for 7 days. No benefit has been demonstrated if treatment with antivirals is delayed more than 4 days after the onset of symptoms.

Surgical decompression of the facial nerve may be considered for patients who have persistent loss of function (ie, >90% loss on ENG at 2 weeks). This degree of degeneration of the facial nerve appears to be irreversible after 2 to 3 weeks. Patients may have several complications from facial nerve decompression, including permanent unilateral deafness.[16] The role of surgical decompression remains controversial.[26]

Referral to a neurologist should be carried out if facial paralysis is bilateral or not improving within 2 to 3 weeks after onset.[16]

Because patients with facial paralysis are usually unable to close the affected eye, they are at risk for irritation and dryness of the globe, leading to corneal abrasion and ulceration. To minimize this risk, patients should be instructed to use artificial tears several times during the day, use lubricating ointment in the eye at bedtime, and tape the eyelid shut at night.

FACIAL PARALYSIS IN CHILDREN

Facial paralysis in children is different than in adults in that up to 70% of cases have identifiable secondary causes compared to 25% to 40% in adults.[27] Except in areas endemic for Lyme disease, the most common cause of facial paralysis in children is acute otitis media. Paralysis of facial muscles usually begins 5 to 8 days after the onset of signs and symptoms of acute otitis media.

Lyme disease is more common as a cause of facial paralysis in children in endemic areas. Facial nerve paralysis from Lyme disease may be unilateral or bilateral and can last up to 2 months. Painless and nontender facial swelling and erythema often develop before the onset of facial paralysis.[28] **Box 5** outlines the evaluation of a child with facial paralysis, and **Box 6** outlines the management of the child with facial nerve palsy.

Facial paralysis in a newborn has a 78% to 90% association with birth trauma (forceps delivery), birth weight greater than 3500 g, or prematurity. Fortunately, traumatic lesions are much more likely to recover.[30]

Box 4
History, physical examination, laboratory, imaging, and electrodiagnostic testing in the evaluation of the patient with facial paralysis

History:

- Abrupt onset? (favors Bell's Palsy)

- Gradual onset over weeks? (favors neoplasm)

- History of tick exposure, rash, or arthralgias? (Lyme disease)

- History of ear and facial pain, hearing loss, and taste disturbance with facial paralysis? (HZ oticus)

- Recent history of acute otitis media (more gradual onset of paralysis with fever), otitis externa, or mastoiditis?

- Bilateral facial weakness? (favors polyneuropathies, eg, Guillain-Barré or sarcoidosis)

- History of other central nervous system lesions? (eg, multiple sclerosis, stroke, tumor, myasthenia gravis, and often have other systemic neurologic findings)

- Family history of facial paralysis? (consider familial facial paralysis)

- History of recent trauma to ear or skull?

- History of regional skin cancer?

- History of diabetes mellitus?

- History of pregnancy or recent pregnancy, especially with eclampsia?

- History of facial, dental, or parotid surgery?

- Recent infections? (varicella, mumps, mononucleosis, influenza, cat scratch, HIV, many others)

- History of thalidomide, ethylene glycol ingestion, alcoholism, arsenic intoxication, carbon monoxide poisoning?

- History of autoimmune disease? (temporal arteritis, sarcoidosis, multiple sclerosis, periarteritis nodosa, thrombotic thrombocytic purpura)

- History of recent intranasal influenza vaccine?

Physical examination[17]:

- Inspection of ear canal (vesicles, granulation tissue, edema)

- Inspection of tympanic membrane (cholesteatoma, effusion)

- Evaluation of peripheral nerve function of the extremities

- Evaluation of other cranial nerves

- Palpation of parotid glands (tumor)

- Ask the patient—"Close your eyes"—to test upper facial muscles. Failure to close the ipsilateral eye indicates a peripheral lesion of cranial VII. Central lesions of cranial VII occur in the pons of the contralateral hemisphere or above, and the patient has intact upper facial muscles bilaterally and can close both eyes.[16]

- Ask the patient—"Show me your teeth"—to test the lower facial muscles. Denervation of the risorius muscle is indicated by drooping of one side of the mouth.[16]

- Hearing screen (audiometry, tuning fork, or finger rub test) for hearing loss or hyperacusis

- Taste test. Permanent taste loss occurs in patients with lesions proximal to the geniculate ganglion.

- Inspection of orbit for dryness and irritation. Exposure of the orbit from failure to close the eye.

Laboratory evaluation:

- Lyme titer (immunoglobulin [Ig]G, IgM), especially if recently in an endemic area or history of recent tick exposure

  ○ Serologic testing is often not sensitive enough in the first 2 weeks, and patients should be treated based on clinical suspicion. Patients who remain symptomatic for 6 to 8 weeks and are seronegative more likely have another diagnosis.[23]

Imaging in patients with facial nerve paralysis:

- Indications for enhanced MRI and CT with contrast of temporal bone, brain, neck, and parotid glands

  ○ No improvement in facial paralysis in 3 to 12 weeks

  ○ Onset of facial paralysis is gradual in onset (over weeks)

  ○ Bilateral facial weakness (multiple sclerosis, myasthenia gravis, or other central lesions)

  ○ Surgical decompression of the facial nerve is under consideration

  ○ Suspicion of tumor

Electroneuronography:

- ENG decline in facial muscle function is typically seen from days 4 to 10 from onset of facial paralysis.

- ENG is probably most useful when performed within 2 weeks after a complete loss of voluntary facial function[16] when surgical decompression is considered.

- Among patients who have 90% or more degeneration with the first 3 weeks, only 50% have good recovery of facial function.[24]

Adapted from Tiemstra J, Khatkhate N. Bell's palsy: diagnosis and management. Am Fam Physician 2007;76:997–1004.

The prognosis for recovery is based on House-Brackmann criteria (**Table 3**).[31] House-Brackmann criteria apply to both children and adults. The prognosis of a House-Brackmann grade of I or II is considered good, III or IV is moderate, and V or VI is poor. The prognosis is good if some recovery of facial nerve function is seen in the first 21 days after onset.

CRANIAL NERVE NEURALGIAS

Before discussing specific cranial neuralgias, the pain from neuralgia will be described. Neuralgia is a form of neuropathic pain characterized by[32]

- Paroxysmal, brief (seconds to a few minutes), electric shocklike or lightninglike pain that follows a specific nerve distribution.
- No objective neurologic deficits in the distribution of the affected nerve.
- Attacks of pain provoked by nonpainful stimulation (allodynia) of trigger points or zones.
- A refractory period (without symptoms) following attacks; the duration of the refractory period shortens as the disease progresses.
- Attacks of pain tend to be stereotyped.

SUPERIOR LARYNGEAL NEURALGIA (BRANCH OF CRANIAL NERVE X)

Superior laryngeal neuralgia is rare, and the gender distribution ratio is thought to be equal.[3] The superior laryngeal nerve is a branch of the vagus nerve (CN X) that runs

Box 5
Evaluation of a child with facial nerve palsy

History

- Are there associated symptoms or acute problems? (eg, acute otitis media)
- Is there any systemic disease? (eg, HIV, diabetes, immunosuppression)
- Is there a history of tick bites?
- What is the birth history? (forceps delivery, weight >3500 g, prematurity)
- Is there a family history? (ie, familial Bell's palsy)
- Are any other congenital abnormalities present? (Moebius syndrome)

Physical examination

- Careful examination of facial musculature (closing eyes, elevating eyebrows, frowning, smiling, showing the teeth, puckering lips, observation while crying in infants)
- Examination of ear, mastoid region, parotid glands, and neck
- Complete cranial nerve examination
- Otological examination: external ear, external auditory canal, pneumatic otoscopy, tuning fork tests
- Audiometry
- Tympanometry

Imaging studies

- Probably indicated in most cases of acute facial nerve palsy in children
  o Temporal bone CT with contrast if there is a history of demonstrable mass, chronic otitis media, acute mastoiditis, previous mastoid surgery, or suspected fracture of temporal bone
  o MRI with and without contrast of brainstem, temporal bone, and parotid gland

Laboratory

  o Lyme (IgM, IgG) in endemic areas or history of recent travel to endemic areas
  o Cerebrospinal fluid (CSF) examination for elevated white blood cell count and protein level and CSF antibodies (IgG, IgM) to *B. Burgdorferi*

Box 6
Treatment of a child with facial nerve palsy

- When idiopathic, spontaneous recovery of facial nerve function in children is 80% to 90% at 6 months and nearly 100% at 1 year[29]
- Children may be treated with antiviral drugs and corticosteroids, but the evidence is not as compelling as in the treatment of adults with Bell's palsy
- Eye care to prevent corneal abrasion and ulceration
- Acute otitis media: myringotomy with or without tube and second- or third-generation cephalosporin or amoxicillin-clavulanic acid
- Lyme disease: 30-day regimen of oral doxycycline (children 8 years old and older)
- HZ oticus: prednisone, 2 mg/kg/d for 5 days, followed by 5-day taper plus acyclovir or valacyclovir, 20 mg/kg 3 times a day, for 7 days[29]

Table 3 House-Brackmann classification of facial nerve dysfunction	
Grade	**Characteristics**
I. Normal	Normal function in all areas
II. Mild dysfunction	Slight weakness noticeable on close inspection
May have slight synkinesis	Normal symmetry and tone at rest Forehead: moderate to good function Eye: complete closure with minimal effort Mouth: slight asymmetry
III. Moderate dysfunction	Obvious but not disfiguring difference between the 2 sides Noticeable but not severe synkinesis, contracture, or hemifacial spasm Normal symmetry and tone at rest Forehead: slight to moderate movement Eye: complete closure with effort Mouth: slightly weak with maximum effort
IV. Moderately severe dysfunction	Obvious weakness and/or disfiguring asymmetry Normal symmetry and tone at rest Forehead: no motion Eye: incomplete closure Mouth: asymmetric with maximal effort
V. Severe dysfunction	Only barely perceptible motion Asymmetry at rest Forehead: no motion Eye: incomplete closure Mouth: slight movement
VI. Total paralysis	No movement

Data from House JW, Brackmann DE. Facial nerve grading system. Otolaryngol Head Neck Surg 1985;93(2):146–7.

adjacent to the carotid bifurcation and innervates the cricothyroid muscle of the larynx.[33] Superior laryngeal neuralgia usually presents as attacks of lancinating pain lasting seconds to minutes, radiating from the side of the thyroid cartilage or pyriform sinus to the angle of the jaw and occasionally to the ear, more commonly on the left side.[3] A trigger zone is present superolateral to the thyroid cartilage. The painful paroxysms are provoked by swallowing, straining the voice, yawning, turning the head, stretching the neck, coughing, sneezing, speaking, or blowing the nose. During attacks, patients often describe an irresistible urge to swallow. Hoarseness and muteness may occur during the paroxysms.[33]

The cause of superior laryngeal neuralgia includes a precedent viral infection such as influenza; scarring from surgical procedures such as tonsillectomy and carotid endarterectomy, which leads to nerve compression; and chronic repetitive microtrauma to larynx from singing, talking, or swallowing over a long period of time. The differential diagnosis of superior laryngeal neuralgia includes glossopharyngeal neuralgia, nervus intermedius neuralgia and carotidynia, a pain syndrome in which the carotid artery is tender due to migraine disorder or dissection of the carotid. Differentiating superior laryngeal neuralgia from carcinoma of the neck may require laryngoscopy, electromyography and CT of the larynx and laryngeal muscles.

Nerve block of the superior laryngeal nerve may be diagnostic and usually results in temporary relief. Carbamazepine may be helpful. Neurectomy is usually curative.

TRIGEMINAL NEURALGIA

The incidence of trigeminal neuralgia is 4.7 per 100,000 per year in men and 7.2 per 100,000 per year in women. The age of onset is usually more than 50 years of age.[34] About 1% to 2% of patients with multiple sclerosis will have trigeminal neuralgia.[35]

The pain of trigeminal neuralgia is extreme, intense, sharp, shooting, and electric shocklike. It is felt in the skin or buccal mucosa. Attacks of pain are stereotyped[35] and can be triggered by light mechanical contact (eg, light touch, shaving, washing, chewing, contact with cold air) from a trigger zone. Trigger zones are usually very small and located on the face, nose, and lips. The duration of pain is usually a few seconds, but may last up to 1 to 2 minutes. The frequency of pain attacks is quite variable. The pain is unilateral in about 95% of cases.[3,34] No clinically evident neurologic deficit can be found. Attacks are rare during sleep. The V2 (maxillary) branch of the trigeminal nerve is more commonly affected than the V3 (mandibular) branch, which, in turn, is more commonly affected than the V1 (ophthalmic) branch.

A patient experiencing a trigeminal neuralgia paroxysm typically freezes in place with hands slowly rising to the area of pain on the face but not touching it. He or she then grimaces with an involuntary spasm of the facial muscles referred to as tic douloureux, and then either remains in this position or cries out in pain.[34]

Although a definitive cause of trigeminal neuralgia is not known, vascular loops of aberrant vessels causing compression of the trigeminal nerve appears to be an important cause. Demyelination of the trigeminal nerve is a frequent finding on pathology specimens. Secondary causes of trigeminal neuralgia are numerous, including multiple sclerosis, basilar artery aneurysm, tumor, and brainstem infarction.[34]

MRI of the brain is useful to look for plaques of multiple sclerosis, tumors, and vascular compression.[35] MR angiography (MRA) may also be useful to look for aberrant vascular loops.[34]

The differential diagnosis of trigeminal neuralgia is lengthy. Other causes of similar pain are listed with their distinguishing characteristics (**Table 4**).[35]

Carbamazepine is the drug of choice for trigeminal neuralgia. The usual starting dose is 100 mg 1 to 2 times a day, increasing by 100 to 200 mg every 3 days until pain relief is obtained. Most patients reach a maintenance dosage between 400 and 800 mg, although some patients need much more.[34] Patients often complain of drowsiness when starting on carbamazepine, but this usually lessens after several days.

Baclofen may be substituted for, or added to, carbamazepine. It may be used if the patient experiences significant adverse effects to carbamazepine (especially hematologic).

Other medications or treatments that may be useful include clonazepam, valproic acid, lamotrigine, oxcarbazepine, topiramate, botulinum toxin, and acupuncture.[34]

Neurosurgery is an option for patients who have not had satisfactory responses to medications.

GLOSSOPHARYNGEAL NEURALGIA

Glossopharyngeal neuralgia is very rare. The incidence is 0.5 per 100,000 per year. It is usually seen in patients aged 60 years and older.[3]

The characteristic clinical presentation of glossopharyngeal neuralgia is paroxysms of severe, stabbing pain in the oropharynx radiating upward toward the ear. The pain can be felt deep in the throat or ear.[3] The duration of attacks usually range from several seconds to 1 minute. The frequency of attacks is usually several times to several dozen times daily.[34] Paroxysms may be triggered by swallowing, chewing, coughing, sneezing, speaking, speaking, yawning, certain tastes, and touching the neck or external auditory canal. Obviously this can interfere with eating.[3] The trigger zone

Table 4
Differential diagnosis of trigeminal neuralgia

Diagnosis	Distinguishing Characteristics
Cluster HA	Pain lasts longer; orbital or supraorbital; autonomic symptoms
Dental pain	Localized; sensitive to hot and cold foods; abnormal oral examination
Giant cell arteritis	Persistent pain, jaw claudication
Glossopharyngeal neuralgia	Pain in tongue, mouth, or throat brought on by swallowing, talking, or chewing
Intracranial tumors	Other neurologic signs possible
Migraine	Longer-lasting pain, family history, photophobia, phonophobia
Multiple sclerosis	Eye symptoms, other neurologic symptoms
Otitis media	Pain localized to ear; abnormal ear examination
Paroxysmal hemicrania	Pain in forehead or eye; autonomic symptoms; responds to indomethacin
Post-herpetic neuralgia	Continuous pain, tingling, history of zoster; usually in ophthalmic division of V
Sinusitis	Persistent pain; associated nasal symptoms
SUNCT	Ocular or periocular, autonomic symptoms
TMJ syndrome	Persistent pain; localized tenderness, jaw abnormalities
Trigeminal neuropathy	Persistent pain; associated sensory loss

Abbreviations: SUNCT, shorter lasting unilateral neuralgiform, conjunctival injection, and tearing; TMJ, temporomandibular joint.

Adapted from Krafft R. Trigeminal neuralgia. Am Fam Physician 2008;77(9):1291–6; with permission.

for glossopharyngeal neuralgia may be in the preauricular or post-auricular area, neck, throat (tonsil or tonsillar fossa), and external auditory canal. Up to 2% of patients have syncope (from bradycardia or asystole) during an attack.[34]

Glossopharyngeal neuralgia may be confused with trigeminal neuralgia limited to the mandibular division (V3).[3]

The cause of glossopharyngeal neuralgia includes various anatomic abnormalities affecting the glossopharyngeal nerve including tumor, Chiari I malformation, infarction, neurovascular compression by the posterior inferior cerebellar artery, anterior inferior cerebellar artery, or other vessels and compression of cranial nerve IX by a calcified or elongated styloid process (Eagle syndrome).[36,37] Vertebral artery dissection can also cause glossopharyngeal neuralgia.

Application of local anesthetic to trigger point gives relief and may serve as a diagnostic aid.[34] The physical examination is usually normal, except for findings of a trigger point. A plain film may help identify an elongated styloid process.[37] An enhanced MRI may identify vascular compression or tumor.[36]

Treatment of glossopharyngeal neuralgia includes the use of carbamazepine and other anticonvulsants, as in the treatment of trigeminal neuralgia. Baclofen and gabapentin may also be helpful. If the cause proves to be from vascular compression of the glossopharyngeal nerve on MRI, vascular decompression may be indicated.

NERVUS INTERMEDIUS (GENICULATE) NEURALGIA

The nervus intermedius is a small branch of the facial nerve (VII) that innervates the inner ear, middle ear, mastoid cells, eustachian tube, and part of the pinna of the ear.[4] Neuralgia of the nervus intermedius is very rare, with an estimated incidence of 0.03 per 100,000 per year. It is seen most commonly in patients older than 50 years of age,[3] and middle-aged women seem to be affected more than men.[4]

The clinical characteristics of nervus intermedius neuralgia include paroxysms of intense, lightninglike, or burning pain limited to the depths of the ear.[38,39] The pain is occasionally located deeply in the face behind the orbits and posterior nasal cavity. Painful paroxysms typically last from a few seconds to not more than a few minutes. The frequency of attacks is quite variable. A trigger zone may be located on the posterior wall of the external auditory canal.[38] Patients may have a sense of bitter taste in their mouth during an attack.

Nervus intermedius neuralgia may be difficult to differentiate from glossopharyngeal neuralgia confined to the ear. Contrast-enhanced imaging of the brain focusing on the internal auditory meatus and MRA looking for ectatic or aberrant vessels, which may compress the nerve, may help in localization of the cause.

Treatment of nervus intermedius neuralgia includes carbamazepine and other anticonvulsants used in the treatment of trigeminal neuralgia. Neurosurgery may be necessary for patients not responding to medications.[38]

RAEDER PARATRIGEMINAL SYNDROME

Raeder paratrigeminal syndrome is a rare neuralgia of the trigeminal nerve. The onset is usually in the middle-aged and there is a male preponderance.[3] Clinical characteristics include decreased sensation in the distribution of the trigeminal nerve, most commonly the ophthalmic division.[40] Weakness of the muscles innervated by the trigeminal nerve result in problems with mastication and swallowing. The neuralgic pain of Raeder paratrigeminal neuralgia is usually deep and boring and is not excruciating or continuously severe.[3] Patients also demonstrate unilateral oculosympathetic paresis, usually miosis and ptosis, similar to Horner syndrome. Unlike Horner syndrome, facial sweating is preserved.

Other cranial nerves may be involved (II, III, IV, V, VI).[3] The cause of Raeder paratrigeminal neuralgia may result from trauma or middle cranial fossa tumor. Treatment includes surgery if a mass lesion is present. Otherwise, analgesics may control the discomfort.

SUMMARY

Discussion of localized cranial nerve neurologic syndromes becomes complicated due to the many types of peripheral nerve fibers (ie, general and special, visceral and somatic, afferent and efferent) and specialized functions of each cranial nerve. The tortuous courses of cranial nerves through foramina of the skull demonstrate vulnerability of cranial nerves to compression by adjacent anatomic structures. Cranial nerves may be involved in many disease processes. Because most of the cranial nerve neuralgias are relatively rare in primary care, sorting through the differential diagnosis can be confusing and difficult. It is important to recognize situations that require urgent attention so patients will receive optimal care.

REFERENCES

1. Ely J, Hansen M, Clark E. Diagnosis of ear pain. Am Fam Physician 2008;77(5): 621–8.
2. Egala A, Clamp P, Hajioff D. Ear pain and facial palsy. BMJ 2012;345:e6000.

3. Merskey H, Bogduk N. International Association for the Study of Pain. Task Force on Taxonomy: classification of chronic pain: descriptions of chronic pain syndromes and definitions of pain terms. 2nd edition. Seattle (WA): IASP Press; 1994.
4. Boes CJ, Copobianco DJ, Cutrer FM, et al. Headache and other craniofacial pain. In: Bradley WG, Daroff RB, Fenichel GM, editors. Neurology in clinical practice. Philadelphia: Butterworth Heinemann; 2012. p. 1703–44.
5. Dworkin RH, Johnson RW, Breuer J, et al. Recommendations for the management of Herpes Zoster. Clin Infect Dis 2007;44:S1–26.
6. Bowsher D. Postherpetic neuralgia and its treatment: a retrospective survey of 191 patients. J Pain Symptom Manage 1996;12:290.
7. Pavan-Langston D. Herpes zoster ophthalmicus. Neurology 1995;45:S50.
8. Tomkinson A, Roblin DG, Brown MJ. Hutchinson's and its importance in rhinology. Rhinology 1995;33:180.
9. Uscategui T, Doree C, Chamberlain IJ, et al. Antiviral Therapy for ramsay hunt syndrome (herpes zoster oticus with facial palsy) in adults. Cochrane Database Syst Rev 2008;(4):CD006851. http://dx.doi.org/10.1002/1465/858.CD006851.pub2.
10. Uscategui T, Doree C, Chamberlain IJ, et al. Corticosteroids as adjuvant to antiviral treatment in Ramsay Hunt Syndrome (herpes zoster oticus with facial palsy) in adults. Cochrane Database Syst Rev 2008;(3):CD006852. http://dx.doi.org/10.1002/1465/858.CD006852.pub2.
11. Diaz G, Rakita M, Koelle D. A Case of ramsay hunt-like syndrome caused by herpes simplex virus Type 2. Clin Infect Dis 2005;40:1545–7.
12. Adour KK. Otological complications of herpes zoster. Ann Neurol 1994;35:S62–4.
13. Lee D, Chae SY, Park YS, et al. Prognostic value of electroneurography in Bell's palsy and ramsay hunt syndrome. Clin Otolaryngol 2006;31:144–8.
14. Robillard R, Hilsinger R, Adour K. Ramsay hunt facial paralysis: clinical analyses of 185 patients. Otolaryngol Head Neck Surg 1986;95:292.
15. Kanoh N, Nomura J, Satomi F. Nocturnal onset and development of Bell's palsy. Laryngoscope 2005;115:99–100.
16. Gilden DH. Clinical practice. Bell's Palsy. N Engl J Med 2004;351(13):1323–31.
17. Tiemstra J, Khatkhate N. Bell's palsy: diagnosis and management. Am Fam Physician 2007;76:997–1004.
18. Baringer J. Herpes simplex virus and Bell's Palsy. Ann Intern Med 1996;124(1): 63–4.
19. Qin D, Ouhang Z, Luo W. Familial recurrent Bell's palsy. Neurol India 2009;57(6): 783–4.
20. Clement W, White A. Idiopathic familial facial nerve paralysis. J Laryngol Otol 2000;114:132–4.
21. Quesnel A, Lindsay R, Hadlick T. When the bell tolls on Bell's palsy: finding occult malignancy in acute-onset facial paralysis. Am J Otolaryngol 2010;31:339–42.
22. Boahene D, Olsen K, Driscoll C, et al. Facial nerve paralysis secondary to occult malignant neoplasms. Otolaryngol Head Neck Surg 2004;130:459–65.
23. Wormser GP, Dattwyler RJ, Shapiro ED, et al. The clinical assessment, treatment, and prevention of lyme disease, human granulocytic anaplasmosis, and babesiosis: clinical practice guidelines by the Infectious Diseases Society of America. Clin Infect Dis 2006;43(9):1089–134.
24. Fisch U. Total facial nerve decompression and electroneuronography. In: Silverstein H, Norrel H, editors. Neurological surgery of the ear. Birmingham (AL): Aesculapius; 1977. p. 31–3.
25. Saito O, Aoyagi M, Tomima H, et al. Diagnosis and treatment for Bell's palsy associated with diabetes mellitus. Acta Otolaryngol Suppl 1994;551:153–5.

26. Grogan PM, Gronseth GS. Practice parameter: steroids, acyclovir, and surgery for Bell's palsy (an evidence-based review): report of the Quality Standards Subcommittee of the American Academy of Neurology. Neurology 2001;56:830–6.

27. Evans AK, Licameli G, Brietzke S, et al. Pediatric facial nerve paralysis: Patients, management, and outcomes. Int J Pediatr Otorhinolaryngol 2005;69(11):1521–8.

28. Markby DP. Lyme disease in facial palsy: differentiation from Bell's palsy. BMJ 1989;299:605–6.

29. Shargorodsky J, Lin H, Gopen Q. Facial nerve palsy in the pediatric population. Clin Pediatr 2010;49(5):411–7.

30. Falco NA, Eriksson E. Facial nerve palsy in the newborn: incidence and outcome. Plast Reconstr Surg 1990;85(1):1–4.

31. House JW, Brackmann DE. Facial nerve grading system. Otolaryngol Head Neck Surg 1985;93(2):146–7.

32. Goodwin JG, Bajwa ZH. Understanding the patient with chronic pain. In: Warfield CA, Bajwa ZH, editors. Principles and practice of pain medicine. New York: McGraw-Hill; 2004. p. 55.

33. Bruyn G. Superior laryngeal neuralgia. Cephalalgia 2003;3:235–40.

34. Rozen T. Trigeminal neuralgia and glossopharyngeal neuralgia. Neurol Clin 2004; 22:185–206.

35. Krafft R. Trigeminal Neuralgia. Am Fam Physician 2008;77(9):1291–6.

36. Hiwatashi A, Matsushima T, Yoshiura T, et al. MRI of glossopharyngeal neuralgia caused by neurovascular compression. AJR Am J Roentgenol 2008;191:578–81.

37. Bruyn GW. Glossopharyngeal neuralgia. Cephalalgia 1983;3(3):143–57.

38. Bruyn GW. Nervus intermedius neuralgia (Hunt). Cephalalgia 1984;4:71–8 Oslo. ISSN 0333–1024.

39. Mokri B. Raeder's Paratrigeminal Syndrome. Arch Neurol 1982;39:395–9.

40. Merskey H, Bogduk N, International Association for the Study of Pain. Task Force on Taxonomy: Classification of Chronic Pain: Descriptions of Chronic Pain Syndromes and Definitions of Pain Terms. Section II, Part II-16. Raeder's Paratrigeminal Neuralgia. 2nd edition. Seattle: IASP Press; 1994.

Index

Note: Page numbers of article titles are in **boldface** type.

A

Acetaminophen, for otitis media, 13–14
Acetic acid, for otitis externa, 5
Acoustic neuromas, 26
Acute retroviral syndrome, pharyngitis in, 93–94
Acyclovir
    for Bell's Palsy, 140
    for herpes zoster, 137–138
Allergic rhinitis, 34–37
    laryngitis in, 106
    local, 38–39
Allergy, otitis externa in, 6–8
Aminoglycosides, for otitis externa, 4–5
Amoxicillin
    for otitis media, 15
    for pharyngitis, 95–97
Amoxicillin-clavulanate, for rhinosinusitis, 55–56, 58
Amplification, for hearing loss, 27–29
Anatomic rhinitis, 37–38
Antibiotics
    for caries, 77
    for epistaxis, 69–70
    for otitis externa, 4–5
    for otitis media, 14–15
    for periodontitis, 81
    for pharyngitis, 95–97
    for rhinosinusitis, 55–57
    ototoxicity of, 26
Anticoagulant therapy, epistaxis due to, 65
Antigen-presenting cells, in allergic rhinitis, 35
Antihistamines
    for rhinitis, 36–37, 41, 43
    for vestibular neuritis, 123
Assistive listening devices, 27–29
Atrophic rhinitis, 37–38
Audiometry, for hearing loss, 23–24
Auditory brainstem response test, for hearing loss, 24
Aural symptoms, in Meniere's disease, 126–127
Autoimmune diseases
    hearing loss in, 26
    otitis externa, 6–8
Avoidance, for allergic rhinitis, 35–37

Prim Care Clin Office Pract 41 (2014) 151–162
http://dx.doi.org/10.1016/S0095-4543(13)00134-6
0095-4543/14/$ – see front matter © 2014 Elsevier Inc. All rights reserved.

primarycare.theclinics.com

Moving?

Make sure your subscription moves with you!

To notify us of your new address, find your **Clinics Account Number** (located on your mailing label above your name), and contact customer service at:

Email: journalscustomerservice-usa@elsevier.com

800-654-2452 (subscribers in the U.S. & Canada)
314-447-8871 (subscribers outside of the U.S. & Canada)

Fax number: 314-447-8029

Elsevier Health Sciences Division
Subscription Customer Service
3251 Riverport Lane
Maryland Heights, MO 63043

*To ensure uninterrupted delivery of your subscription, please notify us at least 4 weeks in advance of move.

Printed and bound by CPI Group (UK) Ltd, Croydon, CR0 4YY

03/10/2024

01040494-0016